SpringerBriefs in Electrical and Computer Engineering

Control, Automation and Robotics

Series Editors

Tamer Başar, Coordinated Science Laboratory, University of Illinois at Urbana-Champaign, Urbana, IL, USA

Miroslav Krstic, La Jolla, CA, USA

SpringerBriefs in Control, Automation and Robotics presents concise summaries of theoretical research and practical applications. Featuring compact, authored volumes of 50 to 125 pages, the series covers a range of research, report and instructional content. Typical topics might include:

- a timely report of state-of-the art analytical techniques;
- a bridge between new research results published in journal articles and a contextual literature review;
- a novel development in control theory or state-of-the-art development in robotics;
- an in-depth case study or application example;
- a presentation of core concepts that students must understand in order to make independent contributions; or
- a summation/expansion of material presented at a recent workshop, symposium or keynote address.

SpringerBriefs in Control, Automation and Robotics allows authors to present their ideas and readers to absorb them with minimal time investment, and are published as part of Springer's e-Book collection, with millions of users worldwide. In addition, Briefs are available for individual print and electronic purchase.

Springer Briefs in a nutshell

- 50 – 125 published pages, including all tables, figures, and references;
- softcover binding;
- publication within 9–12 weeks after acceptance of complete manuscript;
- copyright is retained by author;
- authored titles only – no contributed titles; and
- versions in print, eBook, and MyCopy.

Indexed by Engineering Index.

Publishing Ethics: Researchers should conduct their research from research proposal to publication in line with best practices and codes of conduct of relevant professional bodies and/or national and international regulatory bodies. For more details on individual ethics matters please see: https://www.springer.com/gp/authors-editors/journal-author/journal-author-helpdesk/publishing-ethics/14214

More information about this subseries at http://www.springer.com/series/10198

João P. Belfo · João M. Lemos

Optimal Impulsive Control for Cancer Therapy

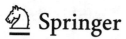 Springer

João P. Belfo 🆔
Control of Dynamical Systems
INESC-ID
Lisboa, Portugal

João M. Lemos 🆔
Control of Dynamical Systems
INESC-ID
Lisboa, Portugal

ISSN 2191-8112 ISSN 2191-8120 (electronic)
SpringerBriefs in Electrical and Computer Engineering
ISSN 2192-6786 ISSN 2192-6794 (electronic)
SpringerBriefs in Control, Automation and Robotics
ISBN 978-3-030-50487-8 ISBN 978-3-030-50488-5 (eBook)
https://doi.org/10.1007/978-3-030-50488-5

Mathematics Subject Classification (2010): 49-02, 49N25, 49Q12, 91B62

This Springer imprint is published by the registered company Springer Nature Switzerland AG
The registered company address is: Gewerbestrasse 11, 6330 Cham, Switzerland

Preface

Designing therapies for patients on the basis of control engineering principles has several advantages. This approach is specially relevant in the case of illnesses, like HIV-1 infection, or cancer, or treatments with heparins, where the drugs administered have a therapeutical as well as a noxious effect. In these cases, control engineering methods provide a systematic mean to optimize the therapy, selecting a time profile of drug dosing that finds the best compromise, according to an objective criterion, between therapeutic and toxic effects. Although biomedical engineering is still far from providing fully automatic "robotic medical doctors", major progresses in computational and sensing technologies, as well as in modelling of biomedical systems, strongly motivate studies in optimal control applied to therapy.

In this respect, one difficulty consists in the fact that most therapies are not applied in a continuous way, but instead correspond to intensive actions of very short duration, such as the ingestion of pills, that are best modeled by a manipulated variable function that corresponds to a train of impulses with varying amplitude. To tackle this issue, most research works consider as manipulated variable the drug effect, which is a continuous function. Although this approach has the advantage of simplifying the class of optimal control problems considered, it has the serious drawback of neglecting the important part of drug pharmacokinetics in the physiological model and is less realistic.

Instead, the present monograph addresses the design and computation of impulsive control therapies. Although the text is centered on cancer therapy, most of the ideas presented are common to other diseases, to which they may be applied.

Chapters 2 and 3 introduce the models that describe the relationship between a certain therapy plan and the evolution of the cancer. Chapter 4 addresses the impulsive optimization problem, including the use of different control techniques. In the last chapter, the main points of the monograph are highlighted and a number of future research topics are suggested.

The intended audience for this book consists mainly of biomedical engineering students and researchers that are mainly interested in cancer therapy optimization, using optimal control and optimal impulsive control, and have a background on systems and control.

Part of this work was supported by project HARMONY, Distributed Optimal Control for Cyber-Physical Systems Applications, financed by FCT under contract AAC n°2/SAICT/2017-031411 and pluriannual INESC-ID funding UIDB/50021/ 2020.

Lisboa, Portugal   João P. Belfo
April 2020   João M. Lemos

Contents

Abbreviations

IP	Interior Point
IS	Immune System
MAC	Minimum Attention Control
MPC	Model Predictive Control
OC	Optimal Control
OIC	Optimal Impulsive Control
PBPM	Physiologically Based Pharmacokinetic Models
PD	Pharmacodynamic
PK	Pharmacokinetic
RHC	Receding Horizon Control
SQP	Sequential Quadratic Programming

Chapter 1
Introduction

1.1 Motivation

Cancer is a general name for a group of diseases that are characterized by a genetic disorder caused by DNA mutations that spontaneously happen or are induced by environmental aggressions. These genetic modifications are inherited and pass to other cells in the cell division process. The modified cells will be subject to Darwinian selection (survival of the fittest cell). Because of this selection, advantages are given to a unique cell (that will give origin to the tumor) so that every tumor is clonal, meaning that they are derived from the same cell (Kumar et al. 2012).

Although the health care industry has experienced dramatic changes during the last 25 years, cancer is presently one of the main causes of death in human populations. Indeed, despite scientific advances led to the discovery of more effective solutions to treat, or even cure, some diseases, mortality due to cancer is still one of the most important problems (Luca et al. 2018). This fact motivates an increasing investigation to find a solution in terms of prevention through regular clinical exams, creation of more effective and less toxic drugs, and more efficient treatments. A better understanding of cellular and molecular abnormalities in cancer cells is leading to a revolution in cancer treatment (Nathan 2007). Some cancers are curable, while others are virtually fatal, the only hope to control cancer being to learn more about its pathology including its behaviour as a dynamical system.

Several articles and reviews (Luca et al. 2018; Urruticoechea et al. 2010; Zugazagoitia et al. 2016), written from the medical point of view, reflect the importance of an approach that envisages cancer as a system, and pave the way for the approach of this manuscript.

There are many types of cancer treatment such as surgery, radiotherapy, chemotherapy, or immunotherapy. The type of treatment that a patient receives depends on the type of cancer and on how advanced it is. Chemotherapy, for instance, involves the administration of a drug into the human body. These drugs are designed to kill cancer cells and, because of that, they also cause noxious side effects, requiring drug dosing

© The Author(s), under exclusive license to Springer Nature Switzerland AG 2021
J. P. Belfo and J. M. Lemos, *Optimal Impulsive Control for Cancer Therapy*,
SpringerBriefs in Control, Automation and Robotics,
https://doi.org/10.1007/978-3-030-50488-5_1

to result from a compromise between killing cancer cells and reducing side effects to the minimum possible.

The above treatment plan is not easy to establish, and arises the problem of how to plan cancer therapies, to achieve the best compromise (Schättler and Ledzewicz 2010). The solution involve modelling and control engineering methods in order to represent the dynamics of the human organism and of the tumor size. Furthermore, optimal control methods are used to minimize the tumor dynamics (Schättler and Ledzewicz 2010). The complexity of the problem increases in the presence of constraints on the toxicity and on the human organism drug resistance. Although much of the published research on applying control methods to therapy design considers continuous control variables, in many cases the administration of the therapy is made in the form of a short term action, for instance swallowing a pill, that is best modelled in mathematical terms as a Dirac impulse function. This type of actuation leads to the consideration of impulsive optimal control methods (Miller and Rubinovich 2003; Arutyunov et al. 2019) for therapy planning, which is the topic of this book.

1.2 Problem Formulation

The main goal of this book is the design of a controller to plan a therapy that minimizes tumor size in cancer, while reaching a compromise with minimizing the therapy toxic effects. This therapy corresponds to the administration of drugs into the human body in a way that is modelled by a train of impulses. To define the train of impulses, it is necessary to define the following parameters:

- the total number of drug administration actions, N, that corresponds to the total number of impulses (therapeutic sessions);
- the drug dosage administered at each session, A_n, with $n = 1, \ldots, N$, that correspond to the amplitudes of each impulse. In a more compact way, consider the vector of amplitudes of the sequence of impulses $A = [A_1, \ldots, A_N]$;
- the time instants in which the drug is administrated, t_n with $n = 1, \ldots, N$, assuming $t_{n+1} \geq t_n$ and $t_1 = 0$, that correspond to the time instants where each impulse is not zero, N being the total number of impulses. It is also possible to define these time instant by the time intervals between them $T_n = t_{n+1} - t_n$, with $n = 1, \ldots, N - 1$. In a more compact way, $T = [T_1, \ldots, T_{N-1}]$.

To plan a therapy, it is necessary to optimize the tumor dynamic response with respect to the above parameters.

Before designing the controller, it is necessary to understand:

- (P1) how the drug administrations is mathematically modelled;
- (P2) the relationship between the tumor dynamics and the drug administration. In other words, it is necessary to define the tumor dynamic response with respect to a therapy defined by a certain configuration of N, A and T.

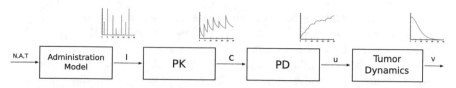

Fig. 1.1 Block diagram of the overall system, including the Pharmacokinetic models, Pharmacodynamic models and tumor growth models

It is possible to subdivide the problem (P2) in three different problems, that can be studied separately:

- (P2.1) how the drug is distributed in the human organism—the models that approach this problem are named Pharmacokinetic (PK) models;
- (P2.2) how the human organism reacts to a certain amount of drug in a certain organ or tissue, and the influence of other subsystems and phenomena (for instance, immune system, angiogenesis, etc.)—these models are called Pharmacodynamic (PD) models;
- (P2.3) how the tumor develops in the presence of the drug.

These problems are connected. For instance, the answers to (P2.1) form the input data to (P2.2), and the results of (P2.2) are the inputs to (P2.3). In other words, it is only possible to study the drug effect on the human organism if the amount of drug that is inside a certain organ is known. The input for the PK models is a signal (i.e., a time function) that models the drug administration, with respect to the three parameters N, A and T. Figure 1.1 represents the block diagram of the overall system, including the block that creates the input signal for the PK model, the PD model, and the Tumor growth model. Figure 1.1 also shows typical plots of the signals at the output of each block.

The third problem of this work concerns:

- (P3) the design of the controller that minimizes the tumor size with respect to the parameters of the signal that modulate the drug administration, N, A, and T. This problem also includes finding the compromise between minimizing the tumor size and the therapy toxic effects that will be formulated as a dynamic optimization problem.

The toxicity sets a limit to the maximum drug concentration in the organism, while the drug resistance sets a limit to the minimum drug concentration in the system. Besides that, the impulse amplitudes generated by the controller cannot be negative, meaning that it does not make sense to administrate a negative amount of drug. So, the controller has, as input, the tumor size and, as output, the optimal parameters that minimize the tumor volume.

It is also possible to decompose (P3) in three problems, assuming fixed and variable parameters. These problems are optimization problems where it is assumed that:

- (P3.1) the time intervals between administrations, T, and the total number of impulses, N, are a priori fixed to certain known values, and the optimization variables are the impulse amplitudes A.
- (P3.2) the number of administrations N is fixed to a known value, the drug administration is periodic with an unknown period T_p (i.e., the time intervals $T = [T_1, \ldots, T_{N-1}] = [T_p, \ldots, T_p]$), and the optimization variables are the impulses amplitudes A and the period T_p.
- (P3.3) the optimization variables are the total number of impulses N, the impulse amplitudes A, and the time intervals T.

1.3 Background Literature Review

The importance of cancer prevention, detection, treatment and management led to an increasing interest in learning and studying more about cancer development. Mathematical modelling has a significant importance in this domain since it allows cancer treatment to be envisaged as a dynamic optimization problem. Tumor size in cancer, interactions with the immune system, toxicity, and drug resistance are the most important factors in planning a chemotherapy treatment, and this is why most of the studies about chemotherapy treatment optimization explore various possible ways of modelling the interactions between these factors (Sbeity and Younes 2015).

No attempt is made here to make a complete state of the art literature review on cancer modelling but only to present the background literature that complements the topics addressed in this book. More exhaustive references in models for cancer therapy design may be found, for instance, in Schättler and Ledzewicz (2010), Eladdadi et al. (2014).

Depending on the type of tumor, different treatments can be used. If it is located on one single area, surgery and radiotherapy are the most common therapies used. If the tumor propagates to other parts of the body, the chemotherapy is more appropriate. The disadvantage of chemotherapy is that it destroys healthy cells, besides the cancer cells, leading to toxicity effects. Because there is a trade-off between killing the tumor and minimizing toxicity, there is an increasing interest in optimizing chemotherapy. So far, clinical trials have been used to plan chemotherapy efficiently. However, due to the high costs and duration of trials, mathematical modelling is now one of the most used tools to optimize chemotherapy (Sbeity and Younes 2015). The importance of modelling is enhanced by the fact that planning therapy is a dynamic optimization problem.

Models range from tumor growth models, such as the logistic or the Gompertz model, to models that relate tumor growth with the immune system, or include interactions with specific body parts, such as the bone.

The idea of applying optimal control to various diseases began in the mid-1970 (Sbeity and Younes 2015). Since then, many publications were made on this subject, for instance Swan (1975, 1984, 1990). In Sbeity and Younes (2015), a review of optimization methods is made.

In order to minimize tumor size in cancer, the relationship between tumor size and the drug administered needs to be modelled. Pharmacokinetic (PK) models describe the drug concentration-time evolution in the body. In other words, using an intuitive expression, the PK model tells what the body does to the drug in terms of absorption, distribution, reaction, and excretion of the drug. On the other way, the pharmacodynamic (PD) models describe the effect that results from a certain drug concentration (Meibohm and Derendorf 1997). Since 1937, PK/PD relationships have been thoroughly studied, allowing the prediction of temporal patterns of drug administration (Meibohm and Derendorf 1997; Paalzow 1995; Welling 1997). With these relationships, it is possible to test drug treatments before actually applying the treatment to the patient. There are many different models used in PK and PD, the most common being Physiologically Based Pharmacokinetic Models (PBPM). Actually, the first PK model described in literature is a PBPM model (Paalzow 1995). In PBPM, the model equations follow the principles of mass transport, fluid dynamics, and biochemistry, in order to predict the drug flux in the body (Campbell et al. 2012). Compartmental models are the most currently PBPM models used, where each compartment corresponds to groups of organs or/and tissues where drug flows and the effect is similar. Depending on how the compartments are connected, there are different types of compartmental models: mammillary model, catenary model, cyclic model, and several others.

In what concerns the PD models, there are also different models that represent the effect that a certain amount of drug has on the body: fixed effect model, linear model, log-linear model, E_{max}-model, sigmoid E_{max}-model and the Hill equation (Campbell et al. 2012). The most commonly used model is the Hill equation, that introduces a saturation effect (Ducher et al. 2008).

Besides drug distribution and effect in the body, mathematical modelling of cancer has been a subject of study for more than 60 years (Benzekry et al. 2014). The interest of studying cancer and the development of cancer treatments is increasing, since treatments have significant potential to enhance quality of life and increase life-expectancies, which may, in turn, lead to considerable economic and social benefits (Luca et al. 2018; Araujo and Mcelwain 2004). There are several different tumor growth models, most of them obtained from fitting experimental data. The most commonly used models are the exponential-linear model, the Logistic model, the Gompertz model, the Dynamic carrying capacity model, the Mendelsohn model and the von Bertalanffy model (Benzekry et al. 2014).

Besides the study of tumor growth models and laws, subsystems that affect its growth have also been the subject of study, like the immune system and angiogenesis (Eladdadi et al. 2014; Urruticoechea et al. 2010; Zugazagoitia et al. 2016; Stockmann et al. 2014; Schirrmacher 2019). The immune system is the defense system of the human organism and its study became very important because of the increased recognition of their role in relation to cancer. In some types of cancer, it is possible to use the immune system in a form of cancer treatment called immunotherapy. Although immunotherapy is not as widely used as, for instance, surgery or chemotherapy, it causes fewer side effects than other treatments, it can boost other cancer treatments (Schirrmacher 2019), and is currently attracting much attention from the medical community (Schirrmacher 2019). Usually, it is not used in isolation, but as a complement that boots other therapies.

The angiogenesis process corresponds to the growth of new capillaries from existing blood vessels (Urruticoechea et al. 2010). This process is very important not only during fetal development but also in tissue repair after surgery. However, the existence of new blood vessels may also contribute to the proliferation of cancer and other diseases (Yoo and Kwon 2013). Recent studies report that tumors can grow along existing vessels without evoking new vessel growth. The new vessels created by the angiogenesis process supply tumors with oxygen and nutrients, allowing them to grow (Rajabi and Mousa 2017). This effect led to the investigation of drugs that can mediate angiogenesis, leading to anti-angiogenesis processes. By adding the knowledge about pathological processes, it is possible to diagnose and treat some of those diseases. Some already published works about the use of anti-angiogenic treatments as stand-alone therapy can be found in Cacace et al. (2018), Drexler et al. (2017), Ergun et al. (2003), and as part of a combined therapy in d'Onofrio et al. (2009).

The previously mentioned processes can be combined in order to create a mathematical model that translates the relationship between drug administration and the tumor evolution in time. These types of models have been widely used in order to study different drugs and treatments like immunotherapy, chemotherapy and others (Schättler and Ledzewicz 2010; Martin and Teo 1994). Thanks to models like these, it is possible to deal with complex physical and physiological relationships using engineering methods.

From an Engineering Control point of view, the goal of killing the tumor corresponds to drive a variable to zero through the design of a controller that generates the therapy as a manipulated variable. The choice of what type of controller should be used depends on the problem formulation. Several techniques may be applied, such as adaptive control, predictive control, or optimal control. It is also important to have in mind that the controller design must match a real scenario. For instance, it does not make sense to administer a huge amount of drug to kill the tumor, since it will also kill other healthy cells. When the goal is to optimize the drug administration to achieve a compromise between tumor suppression and toxicity, optimal control techniques are more suitable for the design of the controller. It is remarked that, although not much explored, adaptive control provides a mean to tackle the high variability found in biomedical processes, in particular in cancer therapies (Teles and Lemos 2019).

Optimal Control (OC) techniques are a set of mathematical methods developed to find optimal ways of controlling dynamical systems (Sethi and Thompson 2006). The problem is formulated as a dynamic optimization problem that comprises an objective functional which will be then minimized/maximized under adequate constraints. The problem formulation must be such that its minimum/maximum corresponds to what is actually wanted. Optimal Control theory is an extension of the calculus of variations that was created after the invention of calculus by Newton and Leibniz. The first problem considered by the calculus of variation was the brachistrone problem, where the goal was to connect two points such that a bead sliding along the curve that connects them moves from one point to the other in the shortest time, under the influence of gravity (Sussmann and Willems 1997). The addition of control variables led to the creation of optimal control theory, a field with many different applications: food technology, environmental engineering, noise reduction, economic systems (Bermudez 2001; Buchanan and Norton 1971), and many others including, of course, biomedical applications (Schättler and Ledzewicz 2010; Swan 1990). Although in most studies the control variables are assumed to be piecewise continuous time functions, in many situations, instantaneously changes of the manipulated variable can occur leading to Optimal Impulsive Control (OIC) (Miller and Rubinovich 2003; Arutyunov et al. 2019; Bressan and Piccoli 2007; Stamova and Stamov 2016). In Meija et al. (2020), an inverse optimal impulsive control approach is considered for Influenza treatment, including the description of PK and PD models. Also in Cacace et al. (2020) an optimal impulsive control strategy is used for an application to anti-angiogenic tumor therapy.

Under some circumstances, or simplifying assumptions, the solutions of the OIC problem may be reduced, or approximated, to the solution of a finite dimensional problem (Pierce and Schumitzky 1976, 1978). This situation is the one explored in this book.

1.4 Book Outline

This book is organized as follows:

- Chapter 2 addresses the Pharmacokinetic and Pharmacodynamic models.
- Chapter 3 describes the Tumor growth, Immune System, and Angiogenesis models used in this book.
- Chapter 4 introduces the approximation of OIC by a finite dimensional optimization problem.
- Chapter 5 shows how to apply the methods of Chap. 4 to design cancer therapy.
- Chapter 6 addresses some relevant complementary issues, regarding the controller design.
- Chapter 7 summarizes the key issues of the book and suggests a list of further research topics.

References

Araujo RP, Mcelwain DLS (2004) A history of the study of solid tumour growth: the contribution of mathematical modeling. Bull Math Biol 66(5):1039-1091

Arutyunov A, Karamzin D, Pereira FL (2019) Optimal impulsive control. Springer, Berlin

Benzekry S, Lamont C, Beheshti A, Tracz A, Ebos JML, Hlatky L, Hahnfeldt P (2014) Classical mathematica models for description and prediction of experimental tumor growth. PLOS Comput Biol 10(8):e1003800

Bermudez A (2001) Some applications of optimal control theory of distributed systems. ESAIM 8:195–218

Bressan A, Piccoli B (2007) Introduction to the mathematical theory of control. Am Inst Math Sci

Buchanan LF, Norton FE (1971) Optimal control applications in economic systems. Elsevier, Adv Control Syst 8:41–187

Cacace F, Cusimano V, Germani A, Palumbo P, Papa P (2018) Closed-loop control of tumor growth by means of anti-angiogenic administration. Math Biosci Eng 15(4):827–839

Cacace F, Cusimano V, Palumbo P (2020) Optimal impulsive control with application to antiangiogenic tumor therapy. IEEE Trans Control Syst Technol 28(1):106–117

Campbell JL, Jr, Clewell RA, Gentry PR, Andersen ME Clewell HJ, III (2012) Physiological based pharmacokinetic/toxicokinetic modelling. Meth Mol Biol 929:439–99

d'Onofrio A, Ledzewicz U, Maurer H, Schättler H (2009) On optimal delivery of combination therapy for tumors. Math Biosci 222(1):13–26

Drexler DA, Sápi J, Kovács L (2017) Optimal discrete time control of antiangiogenic tumor therapy. In: Proceedings of the 20th IFAC World Congress, pp 14046–14051

Ducher M, Maire P, Goutellu S, Maurin M (2008) The Hill equation: a review of its capabilities in pharmacological modelling. Fund Clin Pharmacol 22(6):633–648

Eladdadi A, Kim P, Mallet D (eds) (2014) Matematical models of tumor—immune system dynamics. Springer, Berlin

Ergun A, Camphausen K, Wein LW (2003) Optimal scheduling of radiotherapy and angiogenic inhibitors. Bull Math Biol 65(3):407–424

Kumar V, Abbas AK, Aster, JC (2012) Robbins basic pathology, 9th edn. Elsevier Saunders, Philadelphia

Luca F, Salvatore S, Massimo L (2018) Evolution of cancer pharmacological treatments at the turn of the third millennium. Frontiers in Pharmacology, vol 9. ISSN: 1663-9812

Martin R, Teo KL (1994) Optimal control of drug administration in cancer chemotherapy. World Scientific, Singapore

Meibohm B, Derendorf H (1997) Basic Concepts of pharmacokinetic/pharmacodynamic modelling. Int J Clin Pharmacol Ther 35(40):401–13

Meija GH, Alanis AY, Gonzalez MH, Findeisen R, Vargas EAH (2020) Passivity-based inverse optimal impulsive control for influenza treatment in the host. IEEE Trans Control Syst Technol 28(1):94–105

Miller BM, Rubinovich EYa (2003) Impulsive control in continuous systems. Springer Science+Business Media, LLC, Berlin

Nathan DG (2007) The cancer treatment revolution. Trans Am Clin Climatol Assoc 118:317–323

Paalzow LK (1995) Torsten Teorell, the father of pharmacokinetics. Upsala J Med Sci 100:41–46

Pierce JG, Schumitzky A (1976) Optimal impulsive control of compartment models, I: Qualitative aspects. J Optim Theory Appl Springer 18:537–554

Pierce JG, Schumitzky A (1978) Optimal impulsive control of compartment models, II: algorithm. J Optim Theory Appl Springer 26:581–599

Rajabi M, Mousa SA (2017) The role of angiogenesis in cancer treatment. Biomedicines 5(2):34

Sbeity H, Younes R (2015) Review of optimization methods for cancer chemotherapy treatment planning. Comput Sci Syst Biol 8:2

Schättler H, Ledzewicz U (2010) Optimal control for mathematical models of cancer therapies. Springer, Berlin

Schirrmacher V (2019) From chemotherapy to biological therapy: a review of novel concepts to reduce the side effects of systemic cancer treatment. Int J Oncol 54:407–419

Sethi SP, Thompson GL (2006) Optimal control theory—applications to management science and economics, 2nd edn. Springer, Berlin

Stamova I, Stamov GT (2016) Applied impulsive mathematical models. Springer, Cham, Switzerland

Stockmann C, Schadendorf D, Klose R, Helfrich I (2014) The impact of the immune system on tumor: angiogenesis and vascular remodeling. Front Oncol 4:69

Sussmann HJ, Willems JC (1997) 300 Years of optimal control: from the brachistochrone to the maximum principle. IEEE Control Syst. 17(3):32–44

Swan GW (1975) Some strategies for harvesting a single species. Bull Math Biol 37:659–673

Swan GW (1984) Applications of optimal control theory in biomedicine, vol 60. Dekker, New York, p 1

Swan GW (1990) Role of optimal control theory in cancer chemotherapy applications of optimal control theory in biomedicine. Math Biosci 101:237–284

Teles FF, Lemos JM (2019) Cancer therapy optimization based on multiple model adaptive control. Biomed Signal Process Control 48:255–264

Urruticoechea A, Alemany R, Balart J, Villanueva A, Viñals F, Capella G (2010) Recent advances in cancer therapy: an overview. Curr Pharm Des 16:3–10

Welling PG (1997) Pharmacokinetics: processes, mathematics, and applications, 2nd edn. American Chemical Society, Washington DC

Yoo SY, Kwon SM (2013) Angiogenesis and Its therapeutic opportunities. Hindawi Publishing Corporation 3013:127170

Zugazagoitia J, Guedes C, Ponce S, Ferrer I, Molina-Pinelo S, Paz-Ares L (2016) Current challenges in cancer treatment. Clin Ther 38(7):1551–1566

Chapter 2
Pharmacokinetic and Pharmacodynamical Models

2.1 Pharmacokinetics

In a qualitative way, Pharmacokinetics can be defined as what the body does to the drug. In other words, it represents the steps that the drug takes since the administration until the excretion, called the ADME process. These steps are (Brunton et al. 2006):

- *Absorption*: this is the phase that goes from the moment that the administration is made until the drug reaches the blood flow.
- *Distribution*: in this phase, the drug will be distributed by the blood flow to every part of the organism, possibly reaching the part where it will act.
- *Reaction* (metabolism): this phase represents how the organism reacts to the drug. Only part of the drug will reach the blood flow. This fraction of administrated dosage of unchanged drug that reaches the blood circulation is called bioavailability. Depending on this parameter, the organism will react differently to the drug.
- *Excretion*: in this phase, the drug is transformed in a compound suitable for excretion. The liver and kidneys are the most important organs for eliminating the drug.

The drug concentration variation depends on a variety of factors that are related to the way the organism reacts to the drug, and to the substance properties, as well as to the drug administration method which can be: Intravenous (IV), Constant Infusion Therapy (CIT) or Oral Administration (PO). In this book PO therapy is considered.

Although the availability of the drug is a function of the amount of the drug being administered, it also depends on the extent and rate of its absorption, distribution, metabolism, and excretion (ADME). However, there are some restrictions on the amount of drug that is administered, related, e.g., to the risk of toxicity. The fundamental hypothesis of pharmacokinetics is that a relationship between the pharmacological, or toxic response to a drug, and the concentration of the drug in the blood exists. However, for some, drugs this relationships are neither clear nor simple (Peng and Cheung 2009). Nevertheless, pharmacokinetics plays an important role

J. P. Belfo and J. M. Lemos, *Optimal Impulsive Control for Cancer Therapy*,
SpringerBriefs in Control, Automation and Robotics,
https://doi.org/10.1007/978-3-030-50488-5_2

in a dose-efficacy scheme, providing a quantitative relationship between dose and plasma concentration.

The parameters of a PK model can be obtained by direct measurement or through calculation using experimental data, based on mathematical models. More complex mathematical models may also be used to describe pharmacokinetics.

2.1.1 Types of Models

There are two approaches for pharmacokinetic modelling: empirical and mechanistic modelling.

Empirical modelling relies on evaluating experimental data, made of time series measurements of drug concentration in plasma or blood. Based on the estimated parameters, the PK characteristics are determined for each drug (e.g., the area under the concentration time curve (AUC), elimination half-life or total plasma clearance). On the other hand, mechanistic modelling uses the knowledge of biochemical, physiological and/or physical processes involved in drug disposition and drug response in pharmacokinetic model development to derive the model structure and estimate the model parameters (Pilari 2011). Currently, the most frequent mechanistic models used are physiology-based pharmacokinetic (PBPK) models. Those models aim at incorporating the most relevant ADME process involved in drug disposition and can be used to predict the time course of drug concentration in plasma or blood. PBPK models are usually multi-compartmental models, where each compartment corresponds to predefined organs or tissues, and each interconnection (between compartments) corresponds to blood or lymph flows. Because empirical modelling creates models by observations and experiments, it includes non-compartmental models.

2.1.2 Compartmental Models

Compartmental models are based on dividing the organism into spaces (compartments) with identical dynamic (typically divided into one, two or three compartments). The state of compartmental models is made of the drug concentration in each compartment. Figure 2.1 represents the most common compartment models. In the catenary model (Fig. 2.1a), the compartments are arranged in a chain, with each cell connected only to its neighbors, while in the mammillary model (Fig. 2.1b) there is a central compartment with peripheral compartments connected only to it. There are other types of compartmental models, for instance cyclic models (like the catenary model, but in which the first and last compartments are connected), closed models or open models.

Compartmental models have two important characteristics: mass conservation and positivity. In other words, the compartmental models are governed by a law of mass conservation (that states that for any system closed to all transfers of matter

Fig. 2.1 General compartment model architectures

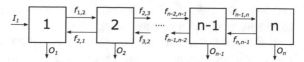

(a) Catenary compartment model

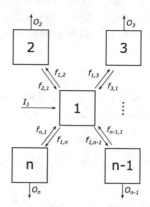

(b) Mammillary compartment model

and energy, the mass of the system must remain constant over time) and its state variables are constrained to remain non-negative along time.

Using the mass conservation law, a system of first order ordinary differential equations for the concentration of the substance considered in each compartment can be written Bastin and Guffens (2006). Each compartment contains a concentration $c_i(t)$ of the drug considered. Grouping all the quantities, corresponding to the different compartments in one vector, it is possible to write the state vector as $c(t) = (c_1(t), c_2(t), \ldots, c_n(t))^T$. The connections between compartment i and j are represented by a function $f_{i,j}(c(t))$ that represents the flow from compartment j to compartment i, and the input (injected from the outside to some compartments) and output (expelled from some compartments to the outside) are expressed by $I_i(t)$ and $O(c(t))$ (Bastin and Guffens 2006). The quantity variation in a compartment i can thus be expressed by the sum of all the inputs from other compartments or from the outside, minus the sum of all the outputs to other compartments or to the outside, plus the initial concentration inside the compartments. In other words, in a general case where it is assumed that all the compartments have connections between them, and that all compartments have input and output functions, the variation rate of the state vector $\dot{c}(t)$ can be written by

$$\dot{c}_i = \sum_{j \neq i} f_{ji}(c) - \sum_{j \neq i} f_{ij}(c) - O_i(c) + I_i, \quad i = 1, \ldots, n. \tag{2.1}$$

The model defined in Eq. (2.1) makes sense only if the quantities in all the compartments remain non-negative along time. The flow $(f_{i,j}(c(t)))$, inflow $(I_i(t))$, and outflow $(O_i(c))$ functions are non-negative for all time (Bastin and Guffens 2006). Actually, it does not make sense to administer a negative amount of drug to a patient, as well as expelling to the outside and transferring to other organs a negative amount of drug. Furthermore, it is not possible to have positive flows from an empty compartment. This last statement implies that, if $c_i = 0$, then $f_{i,j}(c) = 0$ and $O_i(c) = 0$. Under this condition, it is reasonable to assume that

$$f_{i,j}(c) = r_{i,j}(c)c_i, \quad O_i(c) = q_i(c)c_i, \tag{2.2}$$

where $r_{i,j}(c)$ and $q_i(c)$ are defined to be continuous and non-negative for all values of c (Bastin and Guffens 2006). Rewriting Eq. (2.1) according to this assumption, it follows that

$$\dot{c}_i = \sum_{j \neq i} r_{j,i}(c)c_j - \sum_{j \neq i} r_{i,j}(c)c_i - q_i(c)c_i + I_i, \quad i = 1, ..., n. \tag{2.3}$$

This set of first order ordinary differential equations form the state representation of the compartmental model.

Models of this form are used to represent industrial processes (chemical reactors (Imsland et al. 2003), grinding circuits (Grognard et al. 2001), queuing systems (Farina and Rinaldi 2000), and many others, for instance lipoprotein metabolism and potassium ion transfer models (Haddad et al. 2010).

2.1.3 Positive Systems

Compartmental models have many interesting properties that are widely documented in the literature and of which advantage may be taken to design controllers (Haddad et al. 2010). As stated in the last section, compartmental models are positive systems. It can be proved that, if the flow, inflow, outflow functions, and also the initial conditions are non-negative for all compartments, then the concentration remains non-negative (higher or equal to zero) for all time.

The other property is that a compartmental system is mass conservative. In the special case of a system without inflows $(I_i = 0, i = 1, ..., n)$ and outflows $(O_i(c) = 0, i = 1, .., n)$, it is easy to verify that the rate of change of the total mass contained in the system $dM(c)/dt = 0$ (where $M(c) = \sum_{i=1}^{N} c_i$), which shows that the total mass is conserved. Another interesting feature is that, writing Eq. (2.3) in matrix form as $\dot{c} = A(c)c + b$, the matrix $A(c)$ (called compartmental matrix) satisfies the following properties:

1. $A(c)$ is a Metzler matrix, meaning that it is a matrix with non-negative off-diagonal entries: $a_{ij}(c) = r_{ji}(x) \geq 0$;

2. The diagonal entries of $A(c)$ are non-positive: $a_{ii} = -q_i(c) - \sum_{j \neq i} r_{ij}(c) \leq 0$;
3. The matrix $A(c)$ is diagonal dominant: $|a_{ii}|(c) \geq \sum_{j \neq i} r_{ij}(c)$.

An important feature that Metzler matrices imprint to a state model is stability, in addition to the fact that the state variables remain positive for all time. This characteristic can be verified for a second order system by computing the eigenvalues of the dynamic matrix. Considering the state space model $\dot{c} = A(c)c + b$, where $A(c)$ is a Metzler matrix, the eigenvalues p_i, $i = 1, 2$ are computed using

$$\det(pI - A) = 0 \Rightarrow p_{1,2} = \frac{(a_{11} + a_{22}) \pm \sqrt{(a_{11} + a_{22})^2 - 4(a_{11}a_{22} - a_{12}a_{21})}}{2}.$$
(2.4)

From the fact that the matrix is diagonal dominant it follows that the argument of the square root is negative, Hence, the real part of the eigenvalues is negative, since the diagonal entries of matrix $A(c)$ are negative. This fact means that the system is asymptotically stable for all matrix values that follow the three properties above stated (Chellaboina et al. Chellaboina et al. (2009)). Using the conditions in (2.2), the continuous time system state $c(t)$ remains non-negative, for non-negative initial conditions.

2.1.4 Example: A 2 Compartment Model

For the sake of illustration, consider a catenary model with 2 compartments, as shown in Fig. 2.2.

Using the conditions stated in (2.2), Eq. (2.3) reduces to

$$\begin{bmatrix} \dot{c}_1 \\ \dot{c}_2 \end{bmatrix} = \begin{bmatrix} -r_{12}(c) - q_1(c) & r_{21}(c) \\ r_{12}(c) & -r_{21}(c) \end{bmatrix} \begin{bmatrix} c_1 \\ c_2 \end{bmatrix} + \begin{bmatrix} I_1 \\ 0 \end{bmatrix}.$$
(2.5)

Let $r_{ij}(c)$ and $q_i(c)$ be positive constants

$$r_{ij}(c) = K_{ij} \geq 0, \quad q_i(c) = K_{i0} \geq 0.$$
(2.6)

Equation (2.5) can then be written as

$$\begin{bmatrix} \dot{c}_1 \\ \dot{c}_2 \end{bmatrix} = \begin{bmatrix} \frac{1}{V_1}(-K_{12} - K_{10}) & \frac{1}{V_1}K_{21} \\ \frac{1}{V_2}K_{12} & -\frac{1}{V_2}K_{21} \end{bmatrix} \begin{bmatrix} c_1 \\ c_2 \end{bmatrix} + \begin{bmatrix} \frac{1}{V_1} \\ 0 \end{bmatrix} u,$$
(2.7)

Fig. 2.2 Catenary model with 2 compartments

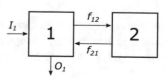

Table 2.1 Pharmacokinetic parameters for *Bevacizumab* and *Atezolizumab*

Parameter	Bevacizumab	Atezolizumab	Units
K_{12}	0.223	0.3	day^{-1}
K_{21}	0.215	0.2455	day^{-1}
K_{10}	0.0779	0.0643	day^{-1}
V_1	2660	3110	ml
V_2	2660	3110	ml

where the vector $c = [c_1, c_2]^T$ is the drug concentration, $u = I_1$ is the input signal and V_i is the volume of compartment i, for $i = 1, 2$.

In this book, the catenary model with 2 compartments presented in (2.7) is used as target model to study the PK behaviour. As stated in the introduction, the compartment model input signal I_1 (Fig. 2.2) is modelled as a train of Dirac impulses, a mathematical entity to be discussed in Chap. 4.

The values of the constants K_{ij} depend on the drug. Table 2.1 summarizes some estimated values for two drugs currently used in cancer chemotherapy, where the volume of both compartments are assumed to be equal.

2.2 Pharmacodynamics

Pharmacodynamics (PD) aims at defining a relation between drug concentration and the effect in the human organism. As for PK modelling, there are also two general approaches for PD modelling: classical modelling (i.e. empirical modelling) and mechanistic modelling (Pilari 2011). In the first of these approaches, the type of the model and the values of the model parameters are derived from experimental measurements. In mechanistic modelling, the structure of the model is defined through the understanding of biochemical and physical processes involved in drug response. In a general way, the qualitative description of PD models are important to establish appropriate band dosage for patients as well as to compare efficacy and safety of one drug with another (Hacker et al. 2009).

The simplest PD models describe the relationship between drug effect and drug concentration. These relationships are often represented by the Hill Equation introduced by Wagner in 1968 (Goutelle et al. 2008)

$$u(t) = u_{\max} \frac{c^\alpha(t)}{c_{50}^\alpha + c^\alpha(t)}, \tag{2.8}$$

where c_{50} is the drug concentration value for which the half-maximal effect is reached and α is the Hill coefficient that defines the steepness of the resulting sigmoid curve (see Fig. 2.3). The PD behaviour depends on the current drug concentration, on the

Table 2.2 Pharmacodynamic parameters for *Bevacizumab* and *Atezolizumab*

Parameter	Bevacizumab	Atezolizumab	Units
c_{50}	72	40	pM
c_{50}	0.1074	0.0578	μg/mL
c_{50}	11.4274	7.1903	mg/kg

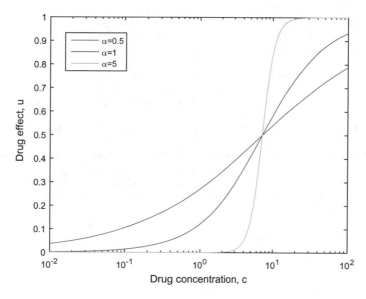

Fig. 2.3 Drug effect as a function of drug (*Atezolizumab*) concentration, with $u_{max} = 1$, for different values of α

drug concentration variation, and on the c_{50} value. Table 2.2 shows some values for this parameter for the two drugs previously considered.

Figure 2.3 represents the drug effect as a function of drug concentration for *Atezolizumab*. As it is possible to see, the Hill Equation introduces a saturation on the effect. For small concentrations, its effect is very small, while for high concentrations, its effect saturates, meaning that higher dosages will not have a higher effect in the tumor. The saturation value is given by the parameter u_{max}.

The above models relate the rate of drug administration to drug effect.

In the following chapter, a more detailed discussion regarding Tumor Growth Models and some subsystems that affect it, such as the immune system (IS) and angiogenesis, is performed.

References

Bastin G, Guffens V (2006) Congestion control in compartment network systems. Elsevier, Syst Control Lett 55:689–696

Brunton LL, Lazo JS, Parker KL (2006) The pharmacological basis of therapeutics, 11th edn. MC Graw Hill, New York

Chellaboina V, Bhat SP, Haddad WM, Bernstein DS (2009) Modeling and analysis of mass-action kinetics. IEEE Control Syst 29:60–78

Farina L, Rinaldi S (2000) Positive linear systems—theory and applications. Wiley, New York

Goutelle S, Maurin M, Rougier F, Barbaut X, Bourguignon L, Ducher M, Maire P (2008) The Hill equation: a review of its capabilities in pharmacological modelling. Fund Clin Pharmacol 22(6):633–48

Grognard F, Jadot F, Magni L, Bastin G, Sepulchre R, Wertz V (2001) Robust stabilization of a nonlinear cement mill model. IEEE Trans Autom Control 46(4):618–623

Hacker M, Messer WS, II, Bachmann KA (2009) Pharmacology principles and practice. Elsevier, Amsterdam. ISBN:978-0-12-36921-5

Haddad WM, Chellaboina V, Huii Q (2010) Nonnegative and compartmental dynamical systems. Princeton University Press, Princeton

Imsland L, Foss BA, Eikrem GO (2003) State feedback control of class of positive systems: application to gas-lift stabilization. In: European Control Conference, Cambridge, UK, pp 2499–2504

Peng H, Cheung B (2009) A review on pharmacokinetic modeling and the effects of environmental stressors on pharmacokinetics for operational medicine: operational pharmacokinetics. Technical Report, Defense Research and Development Canada

Pilari S (2011) Novel approaches to mechanistic pharmacokinetic/pharmacodynamic modeling. Ph.D. thesis, Freien Universitat, Berlin

Chapter 3
Tumor Growth Models

3.1 Tumor Growth Dynamics

Despite its internal complexity, tumor growth dynamics follow relatively simple laws, from the macroscopic point of view, that can be expressed as mathematical equations. Tumor growth dynamics has been the subject of biological study for more than 60 years (Benzekry et al. 2014). The models used for modeling tumor growth stem from two general approaches: descriptive models (empirical models) and mechanistic models (Barbolosi et al. 2016; Oden et al. 2013). Empirical models try to describe experimental data. On the other hand, mechanistic models incorporate the understanding of biological and physical processes and factors such as the structure of the immune system, therapy resistance, among others (Barbolosi et al. 2016). However, in general, tumor growth models are used to test growth hypotheses of theories by assessing their descriptive power against experimental data and to predict the course of tumor dynamics in order to determine the efficacy of a therapy in preclinical drug development (Benzekry et al. 2014). Depending on the scale, approach, or integration of the spatial structure, there are different mathematical models for tumor growth. For focusing on scalar data of tumor volume, models based on ordinary differential equations are most suitable. The Gompertz and logistic models are the most widely used in numerous studies involving animal or human data (Benzekry et al. 2014). They belong to the group of sigmoid-shaped models due to the type of response they yield. Also in this group are the Bertalanffy models (also sigmoid shaped) and exponential models (Oden et al. 2013). Independently of the model used, the descriptive variable is always the total tumor volume V as a function of time, which is assumed to be proportional to the total number of cancer cells.

3.2 Logistic Growth Model

The simplest model of the dynamics of a cell population is the one with exponential growth:

$$\frac{dV}{dt} = aV, \quad V(t=0) = V_0, \tag{3.1}$$

where a is the intrinsic growth rate related to proliferation kinetics and V_0 is the initial tumor volume. In other words, a represents the per capita growth rate. This model predicts an unrestricted tumor growth. In 1838, however, Verhulst considered that a stable population would have a saturation level. To represent this feature, Verhulst modified the exponential model suggested in (3.1) by a multiplicative factor $1 - \frac{V}{K}$, where K denotes the maximal volume (carrying capacity) of the cell population (Schattler and Ledzewicz 2010). The logistic model is thus represented by

$$\frac{dV}{dt} = aV \left(1 - \frac{V}{K}\right), \quad V(t=0) = V_0. \tag{3.2}$$

In some cases, the following generalization of the logistic equation is considered:

$$\frac{dV}{dt} = aV \left(1 - \left(\frac{V}{K}\right)^{\beta}\right), \quad V(t=0) = V_0, \tag{3.3}$$

called the generalized logistic model (Benzekry et al. 2014).

3.2.1 Solution of the Logistic Equation

The differential equation (3.2) admits a closed-form solution, which can be obtained by several methods:

$$V(t) = \frac{V_0 K}{V_0 + (K - V_0)e^{-a(t-t_0)}}. \tag{3.4}$$

For $\beta \neq 1$, the solution of (3.3) is given by

$$V(t) = \frac{V_0 K}{\left(V_0^{\beta} + \left(K^{\beta} - V_0^{\beta}\right)e^{-a\beta(t-t_0)}\right)^{\frac{1}{\beta}}}. \tag{3.5}$$

It is important to notice that $\frac{dV}{dt}$ in (3.5) is convex for $\beta < 1$, meaning that its second derivative is positive, and concave for $\beta > 1$, meaning that its second derivative is negative (Schattler and Ledzewicz 2010). In Fig. 3.1, the logistic model and the generalized logistic model for different values of β are represented. As can be seen, the logistic model has three key features:

Fig. 3.1 Logistic and
Generalized Logistic
Models, with $K = 10$,
$a = 0.09$, and $V_0 = 1\,\text{mm}^3$

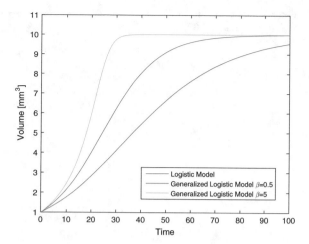

- One has $\lim\limits_{t \to \infty} V(t) = K$, meaning that the tumor cells will ultimately reach the carrying capacity.
- The relative growth rate $\frac{1}{V}\frac{dV}{dt}$ decreases linearly with increasing tumor volume.
- The volume at the inflection point (where the growth rate is maximum) is exactly half the carrying capacity, $\frac{K}{2}$.

In this book it is considered that the output $u(t)$ of the PD model (which corresponds to the drug effect) is introduced through an additional term in the logistic model differential equation:

$$\frac{dV}{dt} = aV(t)\left(1 - \frac{V(t)}{K}\right) - \zeta u(t)V(t), \qquad (3.6)$$

where $\zeta > 0$ is a constant parameter.

3.3 Gompertz Growth Model

As stated in the previous section, Verhulst modified the exponential model in order to create a model whereby a stable population would have a saturation value. Verhulst suggested the term $1 - \frac{V}{K}$, and he created the logistic model. By choosing a different term, the following model is obtained:

$$\frac{dV}{dt} = V(a - b\ln(V)), \quad V(t = 0) = V_0, \qquad (3.7)$$

where a is the initial proliferation rate (which summarizes the effect of mutual inhibition between cells and competition for nutrients) and b is a growth rate that prevents

Fig. 3.2 Gompertz Model, with $b = 0.02$, $a = 0.09$, and $V_0 = 1\,\text{mm}^3$

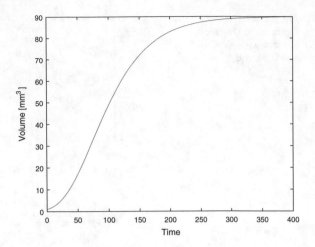

growth for large tumor volume (Benzekry et al. 2014; Schattler and Ledzewicz 2010). This model is referred to as the Gompertz growth model. The fundamental property of the Gompertz model is that it exhibits exponential decay of the relative growth rate $\frac{1}{V}\frac{dV}{dt}$. On solving the differential equation (3.7), the following solution is obtained:

$$V(t) = V_0 e^{\frac{a}{b}(1-e^{-bt})}. \tag{3.8}$$

Figure 3.2 represents the tumor volume evolution computed using the Gompertz model. As can be seen, the volume converges to the carrying capacity $K = V_0 e^{\frac{a}{b}}$.

As for the logistic model, one may consider the controlled Gompertz model, given by

$$\frac{dV}{dt} = V(a - b\ln(V)) - \zeta u(t)V(t), \tag{3.9}$$

where $\zeta > 0$ and u is the drug effect.

3.4 Interacting Subsystems

This section addresses the issue of modeling subsystems that have important interactions with tumor growth. Those subsystems are the immune system and the angiogenesis process. These subsystems affect the parameters of the tumor growth models previously described, which become functions of the state variables associated with them.

3.4.1 Immune System

The immune system (IS) is an internal mechanism of the human body that responds to infections. It is a collection of cells and molecules that are responsible for the organism's defense against a wide range of microorganisms in the environment (Kumar et al. 2013; Janeway et al. 2001; Eladdadi et al. 2014). In order to fulfill this function, it needs to be able to detect a wide range of agents while distinguishing them from healthy tissue (Schattler and Ledzewicz 2010). It includes an innate immunity that is composed of cells and proteins that are immediately available to defend the organism against a wide range of pathogens (Kumar et al. 2013). It also includes an adaptive immunity subsystem that responds (or adapts) to the presence of particular infectious microorganisms, generating a powerful mechanism to neutralize and eliminate them. An understanding of the IS allowed the creation of laboratory-produced drugs to treat diseases. Immunotherapy is based on these drugs, which instead of targeting cancer cells directly, enhance the intrinsic capability of the patient's IS to combat cancer.

There are two types of adaptive immunity: humoral immunity, comprising antibodies that are produced by lymphocytes B (also called B cells, because they are produced by the bone marrow), and cellular immunity, comprising lymphocytes T (also called T cells, because they become mature at the thymus). The antibodies protect the organism against extracellular microorganisms in the blood and tissues. On the other hand, the T cells are important in the defense against intracellular microorganisms. They act directly by killing infectious cells or activating phagocytes to kill ingested microorganisms (Kumar et al. 2013; Janeway et al. 2001).

When the IS is malfunctioning, the mechanisms that are involved in the patient's defense cause injury to tissues and diseases. It is thus important to maintain a balanced immune system.

The competitive interaction between the immune system and cancer cells is complex and involves nonlinear dynamics (Eladdadi et al. 2014). However, there are studies that show that cancer therapy is needed only until the immune system is able to kill the rest of the cancer, and other studies show that adaptive immunity can maintain occult cancer in an equilibrium state (Schattler and Ledzewicz 2010). The existence of such studies led to the development of a mathematical description for the tumor–immune system interaction. The simplest model was presented by Stepanova in 1980 (Schattler and Ledzewicz 2010), and it has the following form:

$$\begin{cases} \dot{V}(t) = \xi V F(V) - \theta V r, \\ \dot{r}(t) = \alpha(1 - \beta V)Vr + \gamma - \delta r, \end{cases} \tag{3.10}$$

where V is the tumor volume, r is the immunocompetent cell densities related to various types of immune cells (T-cells) activated during the reaction (Schattler and Ledzewicz 2010), and ξ, θ, α, β, γ, and δ are constant coefficients. In the original research, an exponential model was used for $F_E(V) = 1$. Other works use a logistic model $F_L(V) = 1 - (\frac{V}{K})$, a generalized logistic model $F_{GL}(V) = 1 - (\frac{V}{K})^\beta$, or even a Gompertz model $F_G(V) = -\ln(\frac{V}{K})$ (Schattler and Ledzewicz 2010). Depending on the parameter values, the dynamical system represented in (3.10) can exhibit a wide range of behaviors, for instance the above-mentioned example in which the adaptive immunity is able to keep the cancer volume so small that it is almost undetectable.

There are more detailed models of the IS that imply a state with more variables and consequently, an increased computational load when one is designing the optimal control (Eladdadi et al. 2014; Eftimie et al. 2011; de Pillis et al. 2006).

3.4.2 Angiogenesis

Angiogenesis is a physical process in which new blood vessels are formed from preexisting vessels. The importance of this phenomenon is that in some works it was observed that tumors can develop their own vasculature. In fact, the tumor stimulates and inhibits the growth of endothelial cells that form the linings of the blood vessels and capillaries that define their vasculature (Schattler and Ledzewicz 2010; Garber 2014). Although those processes are complex, there are antiangiogenic treatments that modulate the growth of the network of vessels in order to control the tumor growth. It is suggested that instead of fighting the rapidly duplicating and mutating cancer cells, the antiangiogenic treatment targets the endothelial cells that form the walls of blood vessels.

The fact that there is no limiting resistance of cancer cells to angiogenic inhibitors could suggest that antiangiogenic treatment is preferable to others. However, this treatment only limits the tumor support mechanism without killing it. Thus, antiangiogenic treatment is not effective enough as a stand-alone treatment to treat cancer (Schattler and Ledzewicz 2010; Garber 2014), but it can be advantageous if combined with other treatments such as chemotherapy, for instance.

There is a simple mathematical model that describes the vascular phase of tumor growth. This model introduces the concept of varying carrying capacity $q(t)$ defined as the tumor size that is sustainable by the existence of the vascular network. This model reads

$$
\begin{cases}
\dot{V}(t) = V F\left(\frac{V}{q}\right) \\
\dot{q}(t) = S(V, q) - I(V, q),
\end{cases}
\tag{3.11}
$$

where $S(V, q)$ represents stimulatory effects and $I(V, 1)$ represents inhibitory effects (Schattler and Ledzewicz 2010; Hahnfeldt et al. 1999). Together, they represent a balance of the dynamics of $q(t)$.

3.5 Global Model

Figure 3.3 shows a block diagram of the overall system that incorporates the blocks previously described. The shapes of typical signals are sketched at the input and output of each block.

In this figure, the first block corresponds to the pharmacokinetic model, more specifically the two-compartment model studied in Sect. 2.1.4, with *Bevacizumab* the input drug. The second block is the pharmacodynamic model, described by the Hill equation studied in Sect. 2.2, where c is the concentration in the effect compartment and u is the drug effect. The last three blocks correspond to the logistic equation, studied in Sect. 3.2, and the immune system and angiogenesis process studied in the previous sections.

The inputs of this system are three parameters: the number of administrations N, drug dosages A, and time intervals between administrations T, as defined in Sect. 1.2. The output is the tumor volume, given by the logistic equation. The parameters used in each block are described in Table 3.1. We note that the nonlinearity of this system is given by the Hill equation and the logistic equation.

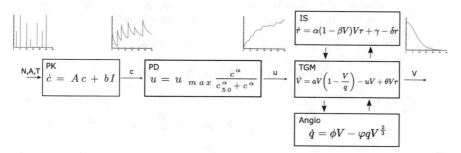

Fig. 3.3 Block diagram of the cancer therapy model: pharmacokinetics (PK), pharmacodynamics (PD), logistic model (TGM), immune system (IS), and angiogenesis (Angio)

Table 3.1 Parameters of each block used in simulations

Block	Parameter	Value	Unit	Range
PK	K_{12}	0.223	day^{-1}	–
	K_{21}	0.215	day^{-1}	–
	K_{10}	0.0779	day^{-1}	–
PD	c_{50}	11.4274	mg/kg	–
	u_{max}	1	–	[0.5; 1.5]
	α	1	–	[0.5; 1.5]
Logistic model	a	0.1	–	[0; 0.1]
	K	5	mm^3	[0; 10]
	$V_i = V(0)$	1	mm^3	[0.1; 10]

The value of the parameters indicated in Table 3.1 are nominal ones, used for illustration purposes. It is emphasized that a major issue in biomedical systems control is interpersonal variability.

References

Barbolosi D, Ciccolini J, Lacarelle B, Barlési F, Andrée N (2016) Computational oncology mathematical modelling of drug regimens for precision medicine. Nat Rev Clin Oncol 13(4):242–254

Benzekry S, Lamont C, Beheshti A, Tracz A, Ebos JML, Hlatky L, Hahnfeldt P (2014) Classical mathematica models for description and prediction of experimental tumor growth. PLOS Comput Biol 10(8):e1003800

de Pillis LG, Gu W, Radunskaya AE (2006) Mixed immunotherapy and chemotherapy of tumors: modeling, applications and biological interpretations. J Theor Biol 238(4):841–862

Eftimie R, Bramson JL, Earn DJ (2011) Interactions between the immune system and cancer: a brief review of non-spatial mathematical models. Bull Math Biol 73(1):2–32

Eladdadi A, Kim P, Mallet D (eds) (2014) Mathematical models of tumor-immune system dynamics. Springer, Berlin

Garber K (2014) Promising early results for immunotherapy-antiangiogenesis combination. J Natl Cancer Inst 106(11)

Hahnfeldt P, Panigrahy D, Folkman J, Hlatky L (1999) Tumor development under angiogenic signalling: a dynamical theory of tumor growth, treatment response, and postvascular dormancy. Cancer Res 59:4770–4775

Janeway CA, Travers P, Walport M, Shlomchik MJ (2001) Immunobiology, 5th edn. Garland Science, New York. ISBN:100-8153-3642-X

Kumar V, Abbas AK, Aster JC (2013) The future of modern genomics, 9th edn. Saunders, Philadelphia

Oden JT, Prudencio EE, Hawkins-Daarud A (2013) Selection and assessment of phenomenological models of tumor growth. Math Models Methods Appl Sci 23(07):1309–1338

Schattler H, Ledzewicz U (2010) Optimal control for mathematical models of cancer therapies. Springer, Berlin

Chapter 4
Optimal Impulsive Control

4.1 Distributions

Control variables that vary continuously, or with isolated finite jumps (such as a square wave), can be represented in mathematical terms by continuous or piecewise continuous functions that to each time t associate a control value $u(t)$. However, even in this case, the actuator actually applies to the system to be controlled an average of the control, given by

$$\int_0^\infty u(\delta)\varphi(\delta)\,dt, \tag{4.1}$$

where φ is a continuous function that is "concentrated" near the time instant at which the control action is applied and satisfies

$$\varphi(t) \geq 0, \quad \forall_t, \tag{4.2}$$

and

$$\int_{-\infty}^\infty \varphi(t)\,dt = 1, \tag{4.3}$$

in order for (4.1) to yield an average. The expression (4.1) defines a linear map that transforms functions φ on elements of real numbers $\mathbb{R}$ and that can be used to define generalized functions (Schwartz 1995, Strichartz 2008).

The function φ on (4.1) is called a *test function*. Test functions are a key element for the rigorous definition of generalized functions and must be defined in an open set Ω. For the purposes of this book, it is sufficient to take $\Omega = \mathbb{R}$. Depending on the choice of the set of test functions, different definitions of generalized functions arise. The class $\mathscr{D}(\Omega)$ was introduced by Laurent Schwartz and is appropriate to the objectives pursued hereinafter.

The *class of test functions* $\mathscr{D}(\Omega)$ consists of all functions φ defined in $\mathbb{R}$ that have continuous derivatives of all orders and that vanish outside a bounded subset of $\mathbb{R}$.

© The Author(s), under exclusive license to Springer Nature Switzerland AG 2021
J. P. Belfo and J. M. Lemos, *Optimal Impulsive Control for Cancer Therapy*,
SpringerBriefs in Control, Automation and Robotics,
https://doi.org/10.1007/978-3-030-50488-5_4

The generalized functions defined using $\mathscr{D}(\Omega)$ are called *distributions*. A *distribution* f is a continuous linear functional defined on $\mathscr{D}(\mathbb{R})$ that maps $\varphi \in \mathscr{D}(\mathbb{R})$ to $\mathbb{R}$ and is denoted by

$$\langle f, \varphi \rangle, \tag{4.4}$$

with φ a *test function*.

Since the functional $\langle f, \cdot \rangle$ is linear, it satisfies

$$\alpha_1 \langle f, \varphi_1 \rangle + \alpha_2 \langle f, \varphi_2 \rangle = \langle f, \alpha_1 \varphi_1 + \alpha_2 \varphi_2 \rangle, \tag{4.5}$$

where $\varphi_1, \varphi_2 \in \mathscr{D}(\mathbb{R})$ and $\alpha_1, \alpha_2 \in \mathbb{R}$. One way to define this functional is by (4.1), with a suitable definition of the integral.

Every function f may also be considered a distribution by setting

$$\langle f, \varphi \rangle = \int_{-\infty}^{\infty} f(t)\varphi(t)\, dt, \tag{4.6}$$

provided that the integral is absolutely convergent. The set of functions that yield distributions in this sense comprises piecewise continuous functions with finite jumps, such as step functions. Therefore, in an intuitive sense, the distributions are generalized functions in the sense that they comprise "ordinary" functions as well as other mathematical entities.

An example of a distribution that is not a function is the Dirac δ impulse, defined as a distribution that satisfies

$$\langle \delta, \varphi \rangle = \varphi(0) \tag{4.7}$$

or, with a suitable definition of the integral,

$$\int_{-\infty}^{\infty} \delta(t)\varphi(t)\, dt = \varphi(0). \tag{4.8}$$

From known distributions one may define new ones by adding and subtracting them, or multiplying by real constants (a consequence of the linearity of the functional $\langle f, \cdot \rangle$), or by scaling or shifting the time scale. An important case, which will be used in the sequel, is the shifted impulse, defined by

$$\int_{-\infty}^{\infty} \delta(t - t_0)\varphi(t)\, dt = \varphi(t_0). \tag{4.9}$$

By combining multiple shifted impulses in a linear combination, the impulse train

$$\sum_{i=1}^{N} A_i \delta(t - t_i) \tag{4.10}$$

is obtained, which consists of N impulses of "amplitude" A_i at times $t_i, i = 1, \ldots, N$. This distribution will be of prime importance in what follows.

However, it is impossible to define the product of two arbitrary distributions (Schwartz 1998, 116–147). The difficulty stems from the fact that according to the definitions given above, a distribution is a measurable function over any compact set (in this case, a time interval), and the product of two measurable functions is not necessarily measurable. Although there are ways to circumvent this problem, the simplest one is based on changing the definition of generalized function, for instance as done in Egorov (1990). Although this subject is quite important for impulsive differential equations that have a nonlinear dependence on the forcing term (the external impulsive input), it will not be pursued further here, because in the model considered, the external impulsive input is assumed to affect the state equation in a linear way.

Another way to generate distributions is through differentiation, a topic that also has an impact on impulsive differential equations. Using integration by parts and the fact that the test function φ vanishes at $\pm\infty$ and is differentiable yields

$$\int_{-\infty}^{\infty} f'(t)\varphi(t)dt = -\int_{-\infty}^{\infty} f(t)\varphi'(t)\, dt, \qquad (4.11)$$

where the prime denotes the derivative. This equality makes sense even if f is a distribution (Schwartz 1998, 33–62), thereby justifying the definition of the derivative of the distribution f as a distribution f' that satisfies

$$\langle f', \varphi \rangle = -\langle f, \varphi' \rangle. \qquad (4.12)$$

For instance, the derivative of the Dirac δ satisfies

$$\int_{-\infty}^{\infty} \delta'(t)\varphi(t)\, dt = \int_{-\infty}^{\infty} \delta(t)\varphi'(t)\, dt = -\varphi'(0). \qquad (4.13)$$

It can be shown (see, e.g., Strichartz 2008) that if the derivative of f exists in the ordinary sense, it agrees with the derivative in the sense of distributions.

An alternative way to define distributions is by means of a sequence of functions (Lighthill Lighthill (1978)). For instance, one may use the family of Gaussian functions indexed by the parameter ε as it decreases to zero:

$$\delta_\varepsilon(x) = \frac{1}{\varepsilon\sqrt{\pi}} e^{-x^2/\varepsilon^2}. \qquad (4.14)$$

The Dirac δ is represented by this family of functions. The sequence of derivatives of (4.14) represents the derivative of the Dirac impulse.

Another way of visualizing the Dirac impulse is through the family of functions

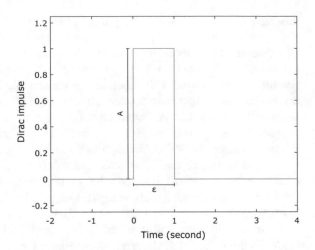

Fig. 4.1 Dirac impulse approximation represented by a rectangle with $\varepsilon = 1$

$$\delta_\varepsilon(x) = \begin{cases} \frac{1}{\varepsilon}, & \text{for } |x| \le \frac{\varepsilon}{2}, \\ 0, & \text{for } x > \frac{\varepsilon}{2}. \end{cases} \tag{4.15}$$

In approximate terms, the Dirac impulse may thus be represented as the "limit" of a rectangle with width ε and height $A = 1/\varepsilon$. This approach is not rigorous, but it provides an intuitive way of visualizing the Dirac impulse as well as a mean to compute an approximation of the response of a dynamical system to this distribution. Figure 4.1 represents the rectangle with $\varepsilon = 1$.

We define the function

$$u(x) = \begin{cases} 1, & \text{for } x > 0, \\ 0, & \text{for } x < 0, \end{cases} \tag{4.16}$$

called the unit step function. This function is discontinuous at $x = 0$. It may be considered the limiting case of the family of functions $u_\varepsilon(x)$ indexed by ε, shown in Fig. 4.2 (Oppenheim et al. Oppenheim et al. (1998)). This fact suggests that the Dirac impulse satisfies

$$\delta(x) = \frac{du(x)}{dx}. \tag{4.17}$$

Using Eq. (4.17), the Dirac impulse can also be defined by the rectangle (see Fig. 4.1) with width ε and height $1/\varepsilon$.

When defining distributions by means of sequences of functions, a crucial issue is to establish the conditions for two sequences to define the same distribution. As discussed in Lighthill (1978), this fact depends on the class of functions considered.

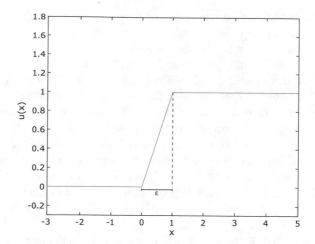

Fig. 4.2 Approximation of the unit step function with $\varepsilon = 1$

4.2 Impulsive Differential Equations

Consider now the nonlinear state model

$$\dot{x} = f(x) + g(x)u, \tag{4.18}$$

where $x(t) \in \mathbb{R}^n$ is the state, with an initial condition $x(t_0) = x_0$, t denoting time, $u(t) \in \mathbb{R}$ is a scalar manipulated input of the control variable, and $f : \mathbb{R}^n \to \mathbb{R}^n$, $g : \mathbb{R}^n \to \mathbb{R}^n$. With an appropriate choice of f and g, (4.18) represents the cancer evolution models considered in this book, which comprise the pharmacokinetic, pharmacodynamic, and subsidiary systems with which they interact (IS and angiogenesis).

It is assumed that the vector fields f and g are regular enough that when u is a piecewise continuous function with finite jumps, the solution of (4.18) with the prescribed initial condition exists for all time and is unique. This statement means that the state x is a smooth function of time that together with its derivative, satisfies (4.18) pointwise.

The situation is different when the input is a distribution such as the sum of time-shifted Dirac impulses such as

$$u(t) = \sum_{i=0}^{N-1} A_i \delta(t - t_i), \tag{4.19}$$

where N is the total number of impulses, $A_i \in \mathbb{R}$, $i = 0, \ldots, N-1$, are the amplitudes of each impulse, and t_i, $i = 0, \ldots, N-1$, denote the time instants at which each impulse occurs.

Since the driving force of the differential equation (4.18) is now a distribution, one has to redefine what is meant by the solution of this differential equation, since this solution can be discontinuous.

Following Bressan and Piccolli (2007) (Chap. 10, p. 234), a control u that is a measurable time function (Vinter Vinter (2000)) is approximated by a sequence of control functions $u^{(j)}$, the limits of the corresponding solutions $x^{(j)}$ as $j \to \infty$ being taken as the solution of (4.18). Of course, for this definition to be consistent, the sequence $x^{(j)}$ must converge to a unique limit x that does not depend on the choice of the approximating sequence. This situation is the one found in the problems addressed in this book, where the dependency of the model (4.18) on the control is linear. Details on the theory of existence of solutions of (4.18), as well as of more general cases, including quadratic dependency on u, may be seen in Bressan and Piccolli (2007) (pp. 241–257), as well as in the specialized literature on impulsive differential equations.

In order to understand what is at stake in the models considered in this book, we integrate (4.18) with the initial condition $x(t_0)$, to get

$$x(t) = x(t_0) + \int_{t_0}^{t} f(x(\tau)) \, d\tau + \int_{t_0}^{t} g(x(\tau))u(\tau) \, d\tau. \qquad (4.20)$$

If the input is the Dirac impulse

$$u(t) = \alpha\delta(t), \qquad (4.21)$$

with $\alpha \in \mathbb{R}$ a constant, it happens that for $t_0^+ = \lim_{t \to t_0} t$ with $t > t_0$, we have

$$x(t_0^+) = x(t_0) + \alpha g(t_0). \qquad (4.22)$$

For $t > t_0^+$, (4.20) reduces to

$$x(t) = x(t_0) + \alpha g(0) + \int_{t_0}^{t} f(x(\tau)) \, d\tau, \qquad (4.23)$$

i.e., solving (4.18) with the impulsive input (4.21) is equivalent to solving the ordinary differential equation (4.18) in the usual sense, with the change in the initial condition defined by (4.22).

This fact may easily be generalized for a train of Dirac impulses as in (4.19). Each time a Dirac impulse occurs, the state is adjusted according to (4.22), and the model (4.18) is then integrated, taking as initial condition this updated state, as an ordinary differential equation in the classical sense, until the next Dirac impulse is applied. This procedure is illustrated with the second-order state model

$$\begin{cases} \dot{x}_1 = x_2, \\ \dot{x}_2 = -2\xi\omega_n x_2 - \omega_n^2 x_1 + \omega_n^2 u, \end{cases} \qquad (4.24)$$

Fig. 4.3 Second-order system response to a sequence of Dirac impulses

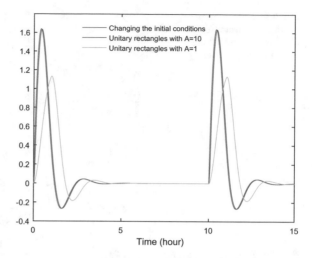

where $\omega_n = 3$ Hz and $\xi = 0.5$. Figure 4.3 shows the response to two Dirac impulses at times $t = 0$ and $t = 10$. This figure compares the response obtained by changing the initial conditions when the impulses are applied to the response to a thin amplitude square impulse of width ε and amplitude $A = \frac{1}{\varepsilon}$ for two values of ε. Although using a very thin pulse yields a reasonable approximation of the response to the Dirac impulse train, it is better, in computational terms, to adjust the initial conditions.

4.3 Pharmacokinetic Model Response

The response of the pharmacokinetic model of Fig. 2.2, a catenary model with two compartments, is now discussed. The state model is

$$\begin{bmatrix} \dot{c}_1 \\ \dot{c}_2 \end{bmatrix} = \begin{bmatrix} \frac{1}{V_1}(-K_{12} - K_{10}) & \frac{1}{V_1}K_{21} \\ \frac{1}{V_2}K_{12} & -\frac{1}{V_2}K_{21} \end{bmatrix} \begin{bmatrix} c_1 \\ c_2 \end{bmatrix} + \begin{bmatrix} \frac{1}{V_1} \\ 0 \end{bmatrix} u, \qquad (4.25)$$

where the vector $c = [c_1, c_2]^T$ is the drug concentration and $u = I_1$ is the input signal defined in (4.19).

Figure 4.4 represents the time evolution of concentrations when a Dirac impulse sequence is applied as input signal. In this simulation, a periodic administration with period $T_p = 50$ days is considered. The values of the constants K_{ij} are described in Table 2.1.

Because there is an inflow directly into compartment 1, its concentration increases immediately due to the Dirac impulse (corresponding to the absorption phase). Through the flows between compartments, the concentration in compartment 2 also increases (corresponding to the distribution phase). Meanwhile, the concentration in

Fig. 4.4 Time response of
the drug concentrations in
the compartments of the
pharmacokinetic model

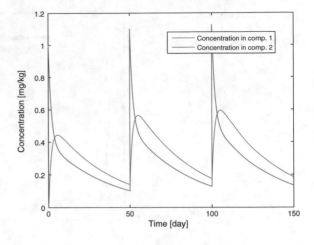

Fig. 4.5 Average
concentration variation
depending on the
administration period T

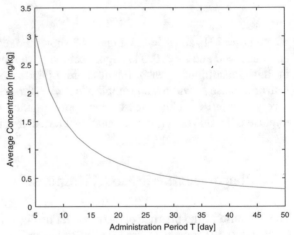

compartment 1 decreases, and a balance between concentrations in both compartments is reached (corresponding to the metabolism phase). Finally, because of the outflow in compartment 1, the concentrations in both compartments decrease to zero, until the next drug administration (corresponding to the excretion phase).

Depending on the period of the administration (i.e., the time interval between consecutive impulses), the final value of the concentration in each compartment, before the administration, will be higher or lower. If there is no further drug administration, the concentration will tend to zero. Figure 4.5 represents the average concentration as a function of the interval between impulses. As one can see, when the administration period increases, the average concentration of drug in the organism will decrease. This fact is due to the constant excretion rate of the organism and will be used to control the therapy.

4.4   A Maximum Principle for Impulsive Optimal Control

The maximum principle consists of a set of necessary conditions satisfied by the optimal control. The original maximum principle (Pontryagin et al. 1962; Liberzon 2012) was valid only for piecewise control functions. This initial result was then extended to measurable control functions (Vinter 2000; Clarke 2013), and in particular, to impulsive optimal control (Miller et al. 2003; Arutyunov et al. 2019).

Consider the following optimal control problem, where the state variables can have instantaneous changes due to impulsive control, which is formulated as

$$
\begin{cases}
min \left\{ J = \int_0^T F(x, u, t)\, dt + \sum_{n=1}^{N(T)} G(x(t_n), v(t_n), t_n) + S[x(T)] \right\} \\
\text{subject to} \\
\dot{x}(t) = f(x, u, t) + \sum_{n=1}^{N(T)} g(x(t_n), v(t_n), t_n), \quad x(0) = x_0, \\
u \in \Omega_u, \quad v \in \Omega_v,
\end{cases}
\tag{4.26}
$$

where $G(x, u, t)$ represents the cost associated with the impulse control, $g(x, v, t)$ represents the instantaneous finite change in the state variable when the impulse control is applied, and Ω_u and Ω_v are the sets of possible values of the control variables $u(t)$ and $v(t)$, respectively. The following maximum principle states necessary conditions to solve the problem stated in (4.26) (Blaquiére 1958). To apply these conditions it is necessary to define the Hamiltonian function

$$
H(x, u, \lambda, t) = F(x, u, t) + \lambda f(x, u, t)
\tag{4.27}
$$

and the impulse Hamiltonian function

$$
H^I(x, v, t) = G(x, v, t) + \lambda g(x, v, t).
\tag{4.28}
$$

Assuming x^* to be an optimal trajectory and u^* to be optimal controls, then there exists an adjoint variable λ such that the following conditions hold:

$$
\begin{cases}
\dot{x}^* = f(x^*, u^*, t), \quad t \in [0, T], \quad t \neq t_n, \\
x^*(t_n^+) = x^*(t_n) + g(x^*(t_n), v^*(t_n), t_n), \\
\dot{\lambda} = -H_x(x^*, u^*, \lambda, t), \quad \lambda(T) = S_x[x^*(t)], \quad t \neq t_n, \\
\lambda(t_n) = \lambda(t_n^+) + H_x^I(x^*(t_n), v^*(t_n), t_n), \\
H(x^*, u^*, \lambda, t) \geq H(x^*, u, \lambda, t) \text{ for all } u \in \Omega_u, \quad t \neq t_n, \\
H^I(x^*(t_n), v^*(t_n), t_n) \geq H^I(x^*(t_n), v, t_n) \text{ for all } v \in \Omega_v, \\
H[x^*(t_n^+), u^*(t_n^+), \lambda(t_n^+), t_n] + H_t^I[x^*(t_n^+), v^*(t_n^+), t_n] = \\
\quad = H[x^*(t_n), u^*(t_n), \lambda(t_n), t_n] + H_t^I[x^*(t_n), v^*(t_n), t_n],
\end{cases}
\tag{4.29}
$$

where H_x denotes the partial derivative of H with respect to x, the same notation holding for the other functions with an index.

The following example, adapted from Sethi and Thompson (2006), illustrates how to apply this principle for impulse optimal control in a situation where the continuous control variable u is not present. This example considers a linear model with exponential growth for a tumor of size x.

Considering $v(t)$ to be the control variable that defines the application of therapy, where $v = 0$ means no therapy and $v = 1$ means a single therapeutic action, the state equation is

$$\dot{x}(t) = bx(t) + \sum_{n=1}^{N(T)} \delta(t - t_n)v(t)[1 - x(t)], \quad x(0) = 1, \qquad (4.30)$$

with b a positive constant.

To solve this problem, one has to find the value of t_i, the magnitude $v(t_i)$, and the total number $N(T)$ of therapeutic actions. The objective function to be minimized,

$$J = \int_0^T Pbx(t)\, dt - \sum_{n=1}^{N(T)} Qv(t_n), \qquad (4.31)$$

where P and Q are positive constants, represents a trade-off between minimizing the tumor size and minimizing the toxic effects of the therapy.

The condition of the maximum principle are now applied under the assumption that T is sufficiently small that no more than one therapeutic action will be found to be optimal. The problem to be solved can be defined as

$$\begin{cases} \max \left\{ J = \int_0^T Pbx(t)\, dt - Qv(t_1) \right\} \\ \text{subject to} \\ \dot{x}(t) = bx(t) + \delta(t - t_1)v(t)[1 - x(t)], \quad x(0) = 1, \\ 0 \le v(t) \le 1. \end{cases} \qquad (4.32)$$

The Hamiltonian functions that correspond to (4.27) and (4.28) are

$$H(x, \lambda) = Pbx + \lambda bx = bx(P + \lambda) \qquad (4.33)$$

and

$$H^I(x, v) = -Qv + \lambda(t^+)v(1 - x). \qquad (4.34)$$

Applying the necessary conditions of (4.29) leads to

$$\dot{x} = bx. \quad t \in [0, T], \quad t \ne t_1, \qquad (4.35)$$

$$x\left(t_1^+\right) = x(t_1) + v(t_1)\left[1 - x(t_1)\right], \qquad (4.36)$$

$$\dot{\lambda} = -b(P + \lambda), \quad \lambda(T) = 0, \quad t \neq t_1, \tag{4.37}$$

$$\lambda(t_1) = \lambda\left(t_1^+\right) - v(t_1)\lambda\left(t_1^+\right), \tag{4.38}$$

$$[-Q + \lambda\left(t_1^+\right)(x)]v^*(t_1) \geq [-Q + \lambda\left(t_1^+\right)(1 - x)]v \quad \text{for} \quad v \in [0, 1], \tag{4.39}$$

$$bx\left(t_1^+\right)\left[P + \lambda\left(t_1^+\right)\right] = bx(t_1)[P + \lambda(t_1)]. \tag{4.40}$$

For $t > t_1$, the solution of Eq. (4.37) is

$$\lambda(t) = P\left[1 - e^{b(T-t)}\right], \quad t \in [t_1, T]. \tag{4.41}$$

From Eq. (4.39), the optimal impulse control at t_1 is finally found to be

$$v^*(t_1) = \text{bang}\left[0, 1; -Q + \lambda(t_1^+)(1 - x(t_1))\right], \tag{4.42}$$

where the function bang$[a, b; Y]$ is defined as

$$\text{bang}[a, b; Y] = \begin{cases} a, & Y > 0, \\ \text{arbitrary}, & Y = 0, \\ b, & Y < 0. \end{cases} \tag{4.43}$$

The bang-bang nature of the optimal impulse control stated above means that $v^*(t_1) = 1$. Using the approach described in Sethi and Thompson (2006), it is possible to find the optimal instant t_1 for the application of the impulsive therapy.

4.5   A Priori Imposed Impulses

For more complicated, and also more realistic, models, the deduction of closed-form expressions for the optimal impulsive control is not possible, and one has to resort to numerical methods to obtain control functions that satisfy the necessary conditions of the impulsive maximum principle described in the previous section. Although such an approach is possible, we will follow hereinafter another approach that consists in the a priori imposition of a fixed number of impulses that define therapeutic actions concentrated in time. First, these impulses are applied at a priori prescribed time instants. In a latter phase, the cost functional will be modified to adjust the time instants of the impulses as well.

It is interesting to note that the application of the impulsive maximum principle leads to postponing the beginning of the therapy. Although this practice is counter-intuitive, it is in line with the results obtained for nonimpulsive optimal control for cancer therapy, when the manipulated variable is piecewise continuous (Fisher and Panetta 2000). Despite being optimal in the mathematical sense, it is clearly better,

Fig. 4.6 Objective function
described in (4.44) for
variable amplitudes, with
$N = 2$, $\rho = 1$, and a
constant reference $r(t) = 0.6$

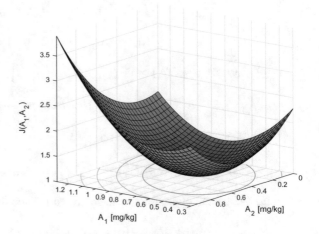

from the clinical practice point of view, to start the therapy as soon as possible, which
can be done when a priori defined control impulses are used by imposing an impulse
at $t = 0$.

In order to explain the approach taken to obtain a suboptimal impulsive control
sequence, an example based on the PK state model for a two-compartment system
is presented. Consider the situation in which there is a certain desired reference r
for the concentration in compartment 1, the objective being that the concentration
in compartment 1, c_1, must be as close as possible to the desired reference, with an
actuation that consists in changing only the Dirac impulse amplitudes. The problem
is thus the determination of the impulse amplitudes A_i that minimize the difference
$r - c_1$ between the concentration in compartment 1 and the reference. Besides minimizing the difference, a term that penalizes the impulse amplitudes is introduced in
the cost functional in order to express a compromise to be met by the drug dosage.
The cost function is thus

$$J = \int_0^H (r(t) - c_1(t))^2 \, dt + \rho \sum_{n=1}^N A_n^2, \qquad (4.44)$$

where $\rho > 0$ is a parameter and H is the operational horizon.

Figure 4.6 represents the objective function described in Eq. (4.44) when there are
just two impulses, with amplitudes A_1 and A_2. In the objective function (4.44) there
are two terms that need to be balanced in order to minimize the function. The balance
is governed by the parameter ρ. As ρ increases, the objective function will give
more importance to the Dirac amplitudes than the difference of the concentration
with respect to the desired reference. For the functional described in (4.44), the
minimum is the vector $A = [0.7097, 0.3715]$. Figure 4.7 shows the time evolution
of the optimized system when just two impulses are applied.

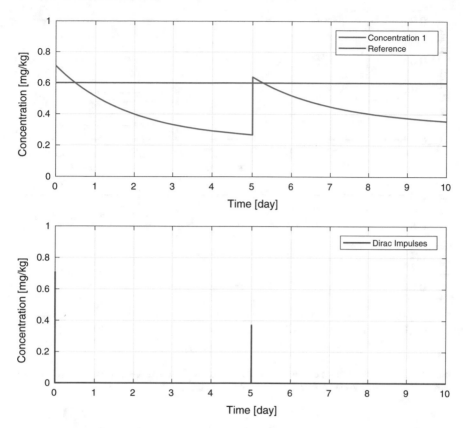

Fig. 4.7 Time evolution of the concentration compared with the reference (above) when two impulses with optimal amplitudes are applied

Figure 4.8 represent a simulation with $N = 10$ Dirac impulses and periodic time intervals with period $T_p = 5$ days. The amplitudes that minimize the objective function (4.44) are $A = [0.7603, 0.4578, 0.3215, 0.2538, 0.2194, 0.2011, 0.1897, 0.1794,$ $0.1648, 0.1362]$. Constraints were added to prevent the amplitudes from being negative. As stated in Sect. 2.1, it does not make sense to administer a negative amount of drug.

It is important to note that if the objective function is convex, then the minimum is a global minimum. A function f is convex if for each pair of values of x, for instance x' and x'', we have $f[\lambda x'' + (1 - \lambda)x'] \leq \lambda f(x'') + (1 - \lambda)f(x')$ for all values of λ that satisfy $0 < \lambda < 1$ Frederick et al. (2001).

If the objective functions are not convex with respect to the independent variables, then in order to find a global minimum, the problem must be reformulated. For instance, the assumption of a variable value for the time interval between impulses may eliminate the convexity of the objective function.

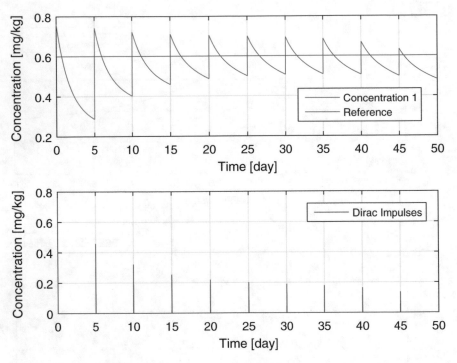

Fig. 4.8 Time evolution of the concentration compared with the reference (above) when 10 impulses with optimal amplitudes are applied., with $T_i = 5, i = 1, \ldots, 10$

In Pierce and Schumitzky (1976b, 1976a) the problem of imposing the drug concentration in a compartment of a PK model is addressed along these lines using methods from linear programming. This algorithm can no longer be employed when the objective is to reduce the tumor size, because the models are nonlinear in this case. Nevertheless, by following a similar approach to the one described above, the solution of the impulsive optimal therapy problem may still be reduced to a finite-dimensional minimization problem, to which methods of nonlinear programming, such as interior point methods, may be applied. In the next chapter, the above approach is applied to design suboptimal therapies for cancer.

References

Arutyunov A, Karamzin D, Pereira FL (2019) Optimal impulsive control. Springer, Berlin
Blaquiére A (1958) Impulsive optimal control with finite or infinite time horizon. J Optim Theory Appl 46:431–439
Bressan A, Piccolli B (2007) Introduction to the mathematical theory of control. American Institute of Mathematical Sciences
Clarke F (2013) Functional analysis, calculus of variations and optimal control. Springer, Berlin

Egorov YV (1990) A contribution to the theory of generalized functions. Russ Math Surv 45(5):1–49

Fisher KR, Panetta JC (2000) Optimal control applied to cell-cycle-specific cancer chemotherapy. SIAM J Appl Math 60(3):1059–1072

Hiller FS, Lieberman GJ (2001) Introduction to operations research, 7th edn. Mc Graw Hill, New York

Liberzon D (2012) Calculus of variations and optimal control theory. Princeton University Press, Princeton

Lighthill MJ (1978) Fourier analysis and generalized functions. Cambridge University Press, Cambridge (reprint from the 1959 edition)

Miller BM, Rubinovich EY (2003) Impulsive control in continuous systems. Springer Science+Business Media, LLC, Berlin

Oppenheim AN, Willsky AS, Nawab SH (1998) Signals and systems, 2nd edn. Prentice Hall, Upper Saddle River

Pierce JG, Schumitzky A (1976a) Optimal impulsive control of compartment models - algorithm. J Optim Theory Appl 2

Pierce JG, Schumitzky A (1976b) Optimal impulsive control of compartment models - qualitative aspects. J Optim Theory Appl 1

Pontryagin LS, Boltyanskii VG, Gamkrelidze RV, Mischenko EF (1962) The mathematical theory of optimal control. Interscience, New York

Schwartz L (1995) Méthodes mathématiques pour les sciences physiques. Hermann, Paris

Schwartz L (1998) Théorie des Distributions. Hermann, Paris (reprint from the 1996 edition)

Sethi SP, Thompson GL (2006) Optimal control theory - applications to management science and economics, 2nd edn. Springer, Berlin

Strichartz RS (2008) A guide to distribution transforms. World Scientific, Singapore

Vinter R (2000) Optimal control. Birkhauser, Basel

Chapter 5
Cancer Therapy Optimization

5.1 Variable Amplitudes and Fixed Time Intervals

In this chapter, the approach described in Chap. 4 to optimize impulsive control is applied to derive optimized cancer therapies. We start by considering the first optimization problem (P3.1) defined in Sect. 1.2, where the time intervals and number of drug administrations are decided a priori and only the impulse amplitudes are to be optimized.

Initially, only the pharmacokinetic, pharmacodynamic, and tumor growth models will be considered. The effects of angiogenesis and the immune system will be considered later. The tumor growth model is of logistic type, the Gompertz model being addressed in a subsequent section. Accordingly, the model used is

$$\dot{c} = Ac + bI,$$
$$u = u_{max} \frac{c}{c_{50} + c},$$
$$\dot{V} = aV - \left(1 - \frac{V}{K}\right) - uV.$$

(5.1)

Figure 5.1 addresses the case in which a constant control action is applied to the patient model and represents the signals drug impulse sequence $I(t)$, drug concentration in the effect compartment $c(t)$, and effect $u(t)$ (see Fig. 3.3), for $N = 17$, $A_n = 3$ for $n = 1, \ldots, N$, and $T_n = 3$ days for $n = 1, \ldots, N - 1$, and $H = 50$ days. The drug effect, given by the Hill equation, is similar to the concentration in compartment 2, c_2, with a scale difference. Saturation does not occur in this simulation. It is important to notice that there is a drug accumulation effect due to the fact that the excretion rate of the compartment model is less than the drug administration rate. This accumulation is important, because the determination of the optimal dosage depends on it in order to respect all the constraints, as will occur in examples presented later.

J. P. Belfo and J. M. Lemos, *Optimal Impulsive Control for Cancer Therapy*,
SpringerBriefs in Control, Automation and Robotics,
https://doi.org/10.1007/978-3-030-50488-5_5

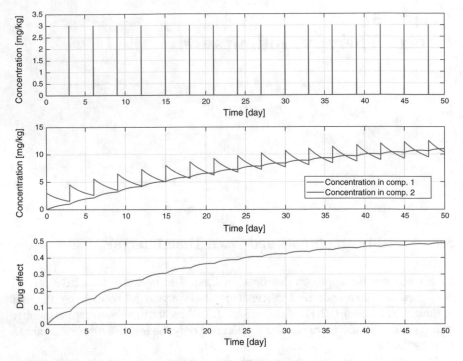

Fig. 5.1 Drug administration $I(t)$, pharmacokinetics, $c(t)$, and pharmacodynamics, $u(t)$

With the drug effect of the simulation in Fig. 5.1 taken as input to the logistic model, the time evolution of the tumor volume is as shown in Fig. 5.2. As one can see, the tumor evolution goes to zero as time increases. For the input signals of this simulation, the tumor size goes to zero relatively fast. If the dosage increases, using the same time intervals, the tumor will go to zero faster. In the limit, if the dosage is very high, the tumor will disappear almost instantly. But such dosages cannot be applied, because there is a limit to the drug's concentration in the human organism above which the treatment becomes toxic to the patient. For instance, if this limit (or constraint) is 10 mg/kg, then the treatment plan described in Fig. 5.1 is impossible, since the concentration in compartment 1 is greater than this threshold after 25 days. Besides the existence of this limit, imposed by toxicity problems, a solution that is more reasonable is one in which the dosage of each administration is not the maximum possible, in order to reduce drug side effects in the patient. So far, the construction of the objective function has to satisfy three requirements:

- minimizing the tumor volume;
- the concentration in all compartments must be less than or equal to some value C_{max}, due to toxicity problems;
- reducing side effects: not choosing the solution in which the dosages are as high as possible.

These requirements will be studied in the next sections.

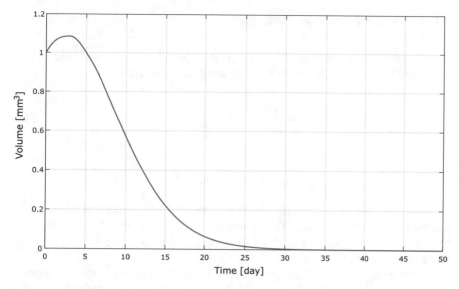

Fig. 5.2 Evolution of the tumor volume over time when the Dirac impulse sequence described in Fig. 5.1 is applied

5.1.1 Minimizing the Tumor Volume

For minimizing the tumor volume, it is necessary to include in the objective function a term that penalizes the growth of the tumor volume. Two possibilities, among others, are

$$J(A) = \int_0^H V^2 \, dt \quad \text{and} \quad J(A) = \int_0^H |V| \, dt, \quad c \in \Omega_c, \tag{5.2}$$

where Ω_c represents the constraints region for the concentrations in compartment one.

5.1.2 Reducing Side Effects

To reduce side effects, it is necessary to add a term to the objective function that penalizes all the Dirac amplitudes. As in the previous section, squared amplitudes or the absolute values of amplitudes can be used. There are thus four possible objective functions, considering the integral of V^2 or $|V|$ and the sum of A_n^2 or $|A_n|$.

5.1.3   Influence of the Parameter ρ

An example of a cost functional that represents a trade-off between reducing the tumor size and minimizing the quantity of drug administered is

$$J = \int_0^H V^2(t) + \sum_{n=1}^N \omega_n A_n^2, \tag{5.3}$$

with

$$\omega_n = \alpha \omega_{n-1}, \quad \omega_0 = \rho. \tag{5.4}$$

This choice yields weights ω_n on the control action that are proportional to the parameter ρ, chosen to be $\rho > 0$, and that grow exponentially with n, where $\omega_n = \alpha^{n-1}\rho$. For N large enough, this choice is an approximation to imposing a prescribed degree of stability (Anderson and Moore 1969).

Furthermore, if ρ is small, the penalization of the drug defined by the amplitude of the impulses is also small, which means that the amplitudes are allowed to have higher values, probably reaching their maximum values, defined by the toxicity constraint. Thus, the question is for which values of ρ the optimal amplitudes do not reach their maximum values. The answer to this question is given by the analysis of the minimum value of the objective function as a function of ρ. Each curve in Fig. 5.3 represents the minimum value of the objective function for different values of ρ, for a specific constraint value C_{max}, considering squared amplitudes and the absolute value of the amplitudes. For this figure, the parameter values $N = 10$, $T_p = 3$, $H = 30$ days, and $C_{max} = 10$ mg/kg are considered.

Fig. 5.3 Optimal solutions depending on ρ, for different values of C_{max}, with $\alpha = 0.9$

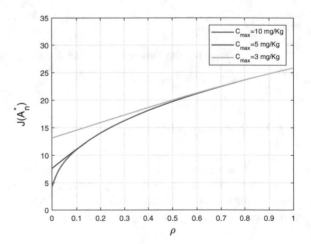

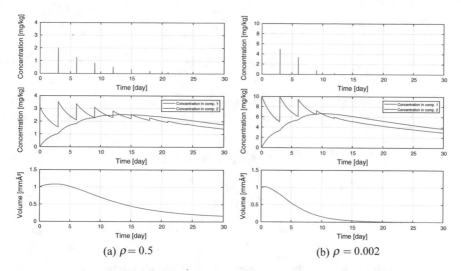

Fig. 5.4 Optimal output signals of administration model $I(t)$, drug concentration $c(t)$, and effect $u(t)$, for the optimization problem 5.5, using a percentage decay with $\alpha = 0.9$, $N = 10$, $T_p = 3$, and $C_{max} = 10$ mg/kg, for two different values of ρ

Several conclusions may be drawn from Fig. 5.3:

- The minimum value of the objective function increases when ρ increases.
- When ρ decreases and the constraint value C_{max} increases, the minimum value of the objective function decreases.
- For $\rho \in [0.6, \infty]$, the three curves have the same value. This means that for ρ in that interval, the minimum value of the objective function is independent of the constraint value. In other words, it means that the drug concentration in the organism is less than 10, 5 or even 3 mg/kg.

Using the information provided by Fig. 5.3, it is also possible to find the values of ρ that satisfy the toxicity constraint. For instance, as stated before, for $\rho = 0.6$, the minimum value of the objective function becomes independent of the toxicity constraint $C_{max} = 3$ mg/kg. So if $\rho \geq 0.6$, the drug concentration in the organism will be less than or equal than 3 mg/kg. The same applies to the constraint $C_{max} = 5$ mg/kg, where now ρ must satisfy $\rho \geq 0.15$, and the constraint $C_{max} = 10$, where $\rho \geq 0.02$.

The choice of the appropriate value for the parameter ρ influences the robustness of the controller. For values of ρ in the region $[0, 0.2]$, the minimum value of the objective function has a larger variation than for the region $[0.2, \infty]$. In other words, if ρ is in the first region $[0, 0.2]$, any small variation $\Delta\rho$ will have a greater impact on the minimum value of the objective function than if ρ is in the range $[0.2, \infty]$.

Consider the control problem

$$\min_{A_1,\dots,A_N} \quad \int_0^H V^2 \, dt + \sum_{n=1}^N \omega_n A_n^2 \tag{5.5a}$$

$$\text{subject to} \quad \omega_n = \alpha \omega_{n-1}, \ \omega_0 = \rho, \tag{5.5b}$$

$$A_n \geq 0, \ n = 1, \dots, N, \tag{5.5c}$$

$$\dot{c} = Ac + b \sum_{n=1}^N A_n \delta(t - t_n), \ c \in \mathbb{R}^2, \tag{5.5d}$$

$$u = u_{\max} \frac{c_2}{c_{50} + c_2}, \tag{5.5e}$$

$$\dot{V} = aV \left(1 - \frac{V}{K}\right) - uV, \ V(0) = V_0, \tag{5.5f}$$

where the optimization variables are the impulse amplitudes only.

In Fig. 5.4a, the optimal outputs of the administration model, pharmacokinetics, and pharmacodynamics, with respect to the optimization problem 5.5, are represented, with $\rho = 0.5$. Note that the tumor volume at $t = 30$ days is greater than if $\rho = 0.002$, in Fig. 5.4b.

5.1.4 Influence of the Parameter H

The time horizon H also influences the optimal solution. In the ideal case, we have $H = \infty$, which is impossible for computations. So the following question arises: how large must the time horizon be in order to yield a good approximation to the solution yielded by $H = \infty$?

There are two ways of describing the effect of changes on H. One of them is to fix the time intervals between administrations, T, to a certain value, and increase H. The other is to maintain a certain relation between H and T_n while increasing H. Figure 5.5 represents the evolution of the objective function's minimum value depending on H, using fixed time intervals (Fig. 5.5a) and a fixed relation between time intervals and the time horizon (Fig. 5.5b) with $\frac{H}{T_n} = 10$ for $n = 1, \dots, N - 1$. As one can see, the minimum value of the objective function increases as H increases.

For the case in which there is a fixed relation between the time intervals between consecutive impulses and the time horizon, the analysis is similar. Note the different behavior of the curves in Fig. 5.5b when $H \geq 130$. This is due to the fact that for the past administrations, the impact of the dosages on the tumor versus their amplitude in the objective function led to very small amplitudes, depending on the time interval. One can see this effect in Fig. 5.6. In Fig. 5.6a one can see all ten amplitudes, and in Fig. 5.6b the last three amplitudes have very small positive values.

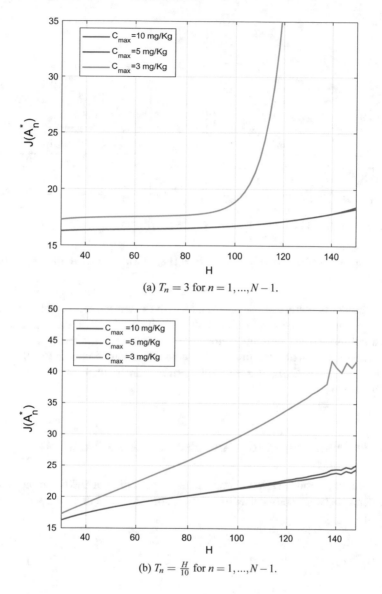

(a) $T_n = 3$ for $n = 1, ..., N-1$.

(b) $T_n = \frac{H}{10}$ for $n = 1, ..., N-1$.

Fig. 5.5 Optimal solutions depending on H, for different values of $C_{\max}$, with $\alpha = 0.9$, $N = 10$, and $\rho = 0.3$

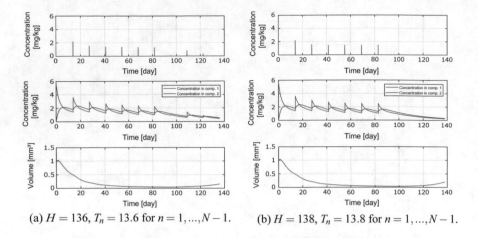

(a) $H = 136$, $T_n = 13.6$ for $n = 1, ..., N - 1$.   (b) $H = 138$, $T_n = 13.8$ for $n = 1, ..., N - 1$.

Fig. 5.6 Optimal solutions for $H = 136$ and $H = 138$, with $\alpha = 0.9$, $N = 10$, and $\rho = 0.3$

This aspect is important, since it tells us that when the tumor volume becomes small, the impact of the amplitudes is also small, and because the parameter ρ for those amplitudes is not zero, the controller prefers to decrease the dosage instead of continuously minimizing the tumor. One possible improvement is to set $\rho = 0$ for the amplitude A_m until A_N, $1 \leq m \leq N$, with m being defined such that there are no amplitudes near zero.

5.2   Variable Amplitudes and Periodic Time Intervals

In this section, besides variable amplitudes, a periodic but unknown value for the time interval between consecutive impulses is considered. Therefore, for the objective function

$$J(A, T_p) = \int_0^H V^2 \, dt + \sum_{n=1}^N \omega_n A_n^2, \quad T_n = T_p, \ n = 1, \ldots, N - 1, \quad (5.6)$$

the optimization variables are the impulse amplitudes A_n and the period T_p. The optimization problem is thus formulated as

$$\min_{A_1,\ldots,A_N,T_p} \quad \int_0^H V^2 \, dt + \sum_{n=1}^N \omega_n A_n^2 \quad (5.7\text{a})$$

$$\text{subject to} \quad \omega_n = \alpha \omega_{n-1}, \ \omega_0 = \rho, \quad (5.7\text{b})$$

$$T_n = T_p, \ n = 1, \ldots, N - 1, \quad (5.7\text{c})$$

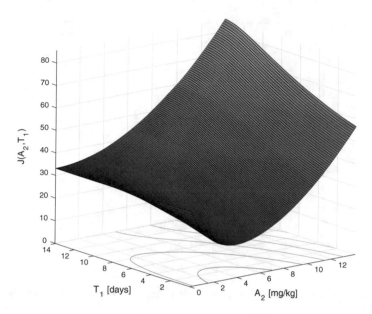

Fig. 5.7 Objective function as a function of the second amplitude and the time interval, for $H = 15$ days, $N = 2$, and $A_1 = 1$ mg/kg

$$T_p > 0, \ A_n \geq 0, \ n = 1, \ldots, N, \tag{5.7d}$$

$$\dot{c} = Ac + b \sum_{n=1}^{N} A_n \delta(t - t_n), \ T_n = t_{n+1} - t_n, \ c \in \mathbb{R}^2 \tag{5.7e}$$

$$u = u_{\max} \frac{c_2}{c_{50} + c_2}, \tag{5.7f}$$

$$\dot{V} = aV \left(1 - \frac{V}{K}\right) - uV, \ V(0) = V_0. \tag{5.7g}$$

Figure 5.7 represents the objective function (5.6) described above, considering only two amplitudes, with the first amplitude A_1 fixed, while the second amplitude A_2 and the period T_p, which also corresponds to the first and only time interval $T_1 = T_p$, are variables.

One can see in the contour lines that the objective function has a minimum value for small values of the time interval. But when the time interval increases, the objective function becomes flatter, for $A_2 = 4$, for instance. These flat areas are problematic, because for initial points there, the optimization methods will not be able to find a good search direction along which the objective function decreases. From some simulations with this objective function and increasing the number of amplitudes N, it is possible to conclude that the function is not convex, because on considering

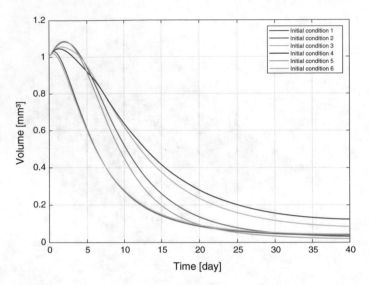

Fig. 5.8 Tumor volume time evolution for solutions from different initial conditions in the optimization method

different initial points (for the optimization algorithm), different minima where found (local minima), which suggests nonconvexity.

Figure 5.8 represents the tumor volume evolution over time, $V(t)$, using different solutions that came from different initial conditions in the optimization method. Initial conditions two and six are the ones that initially yields a faster decrease in the tumor volume. Those initial conditions correspond to the solutions in which the time interval is near zero, in which the objective function presents a lower value. This means that for all the initial conditions considered in Fig. 5.8, the solutions two and six could represent the best local minima to be chosen as the real solution of the problem (i.e., at an approximation to the global minimum). Therefore, the following question can be raised: in a real scenario, is it acceptable to have the periodic time interval near zero? If yes, then the problem is solved. If not, then the next question is how to look for a different solution. One possible answer is to change the objective function (add a new term) in order to penalize small periods T_p. This new term $\Phi(T_p)$ must be a function of the period T_p such that if the period is, for instance, near zero, the function must return a large value so it can change the total objective function in order to contradict the best local minimum.

The function $\Phi(T_p) = \frac{1}{T_p}$ could be used for that purpose, as Fig. 5.9a shows. Another function could be the negative and translated exponential function $\Phi(T_p) = e^{-T_p+\tau}$, as shown in Fig. 5.9b, where τ is the translation parameter. Note that the study of $\Phi(T_p)$ is out of the train of impulses context.

For $T_p \gg 0$, the exponential function presents a greater range of variation than the function $\frac{1}{T_p}$. In other words, for $T_p \gg 0$ and $s > 0$, we have $\left| e^{-T_p+\tau} - e^{-(T_p+s)+\tau} \right| >$

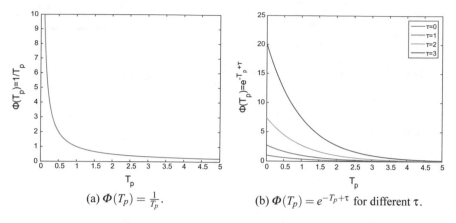

(a) $\Phi(T_p) = \frac{1}{T_p}$.

(b) $\Phi(T_p) = e^{-T_p+\tau}$ for different τ.

Fig. 5.9 Curve of functions that penalize small periods

$\left| \frac{1}{T_p} - \frac{1}{T_p+s} \right|$. This fact represents an advantage for the exponential function and therefore a disadvantage of the function $\frac{1}{T_1}$ in the problem considered. This is due to the fact that if the range of variation increases, the difference between choosing T_p or $T_p + \delta$, in terms of optimality, also increase, allowing the optimal controller to make a clearer choice of the impulse amplitudes and intervals.

Considering the exponential function for $\Phi(T_p)$, there are two parameters to be defined: the translation parameter τ and the weight η that can be applied to $\Phi(T_p)$ in order to tune how much one wants to penalize small periods. The final expression is $\Phi(T_p) = \eta \cdot e^{-T_p+\tau}$. Similarly to the parameter ρ applied to the amplitudes term in the objective function, the definition of these two new parameters can influence the optimal solution to the problem. The parameter τ must be such that as the time interval goes to zero, the term goes to infinity or at least must assume very high values when compared with the other terms in the objective function. So one could have $\tau = 2$. Concerning the parameter η, its effect can be analyzed by simulating the system with different initial conditions for each different value of η. Figure 5.10 was obtained from three different values for η.

As one can see in Fig. 5.10a, when η increases, the time interval T_1 also increases. It is also possible to verify that when η increases, the final value of the tumor volume also increases. This means that when η increases, the new term becomes more important than the other terms, in particular the term that corresponds to the minimization of the tumor volume (the integral of the squared tumor volume), which tries to decrease the time interval.

So far, the weight applied to the exponential term corresponds to a constant value. However, when different initial conditions of the tumor volume are considered, the period penalization may have more or less expression in the objective function. In other words, if the initial tumor volume decreases, then the integral term in the objective function $\int_0^H V^2 \, dt$ also decreases, since the area under the tumor volume curve also decreases, assuming a therapy that reduces the tumor. If the weight applied

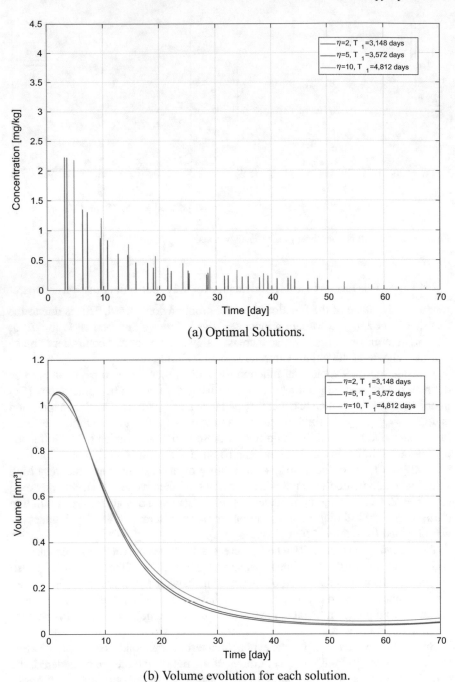

(a) Optimal Solutions.

(b) Volume evolution for each solution.

Fig. 5.10 Optimal solutions and tumor volume evolution for each solution, for $\eta = 2$, $\eta = 5$, and $\eta = 10$

to the exponential term maintains its constant value, this term will always be more important to the minimization methods. So if the initial tumor volume decreases, the time interval will increase for a constant value of the weight η. In order to counteract this effect, the weight applied to the exponential term can be proportional to the initial tumor volume, so the weight applied is $\eta_N = V(0)\eta$, where η_N is the new weight.

Therefore, the objective function when added to the exponential penalty function $\Phi(T_p) = e^{-T_p+\tau}$ becomes

$$J(A, T_p) = \int_0^H V^2\, dt + \sum_{n=1}^N \omega_n A_n^2 + \eta_N e^{-T_p+\tau}, \quad T_n = T_p, \ T_p > 0, \ n = 1, \ldots, N-1,$$

(5.8)

where the optimization variables are the impulse amplitudes and the period T_p.

Besides the penalty functions mentioned above for Φ, there is different function that considers a new parameter T_p^C. This parameter, called the central value of the time interval, corresponds to a value around which solutions for the period T_p will be found. In other words, the goal here is to penalize periods that are far from T_p^C. This can be accomplished by replacing the exponential term with a quadratic term $\Phi(T_p) = \eta_N \left(T_p - T_p^C\right)^2$, where its minimum is in T_p^C. So the objective function expression becomes the following:

$$J(A, T_p) = \int_0^H V^2\, dt + \sum_{n=1}^N \omega_n A_n^2 + \eta_N \left(T_p - T_p^C\right)^2, \quad T_n = T_p, \ T_p > 0, \ n = 1, \ldots, N-1.$$

(5.9)

Figure 5.11 is obtained using optimization methods (SQP) to minimize the objective function. The solution found to be optimal does not correspond to the case in which the time interval is equal to the central value of the time interval parameter. In fact, the optimal time interval is $T_p^* = 4.8049$ days.

In conclusion, when the periodic time intervals are considered to be also an optimization variable, the objective function loses its convexity, presenting flat areas and more than one minimum (local minima). Moreover, on simulating the model for different initial conditions, the solution that returned a lower objective function value (when compared with the simulations that were made) suggests that the optimal period tends to be near zero, which illustrates a situation in which a large amount of drug is administered to the patient at the beginning of the therapy, which may not be desirable. This fact motivates the introduction of a new term in the objective function that penalizes small periods, contradicting what was previously suggested by the simulations.

Therefore, the approach used in this work to find the best solution consists in running the optimization algorithms using, for instance, ten different initial points and then choosing the solution that gives the lowest objective function value. This approach takes a considerable amount of computational time. Each optimization takes about one and a half hours to be completed, which must be multiplied by ten to give the amount of time used to find the best solution (among all ten solutions).

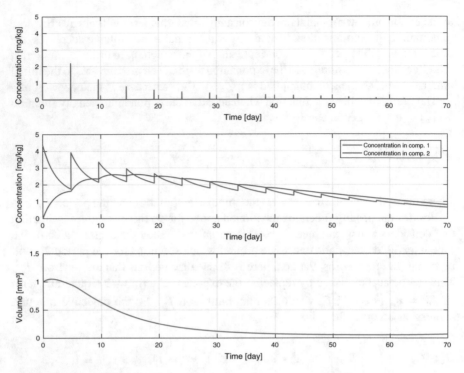

Fig. 5.11 Optimal solution for a periodic time interval, with $N = 10$, $T_p^C = 5$, and $\eta_N = 2$. The optimal time interval is $T_p^* = 4.8049$ days

5.2.1 Influence of the Immune System

As previously stated in Sect. 3.4, the immune system (IS) plays an important role in cancer treatment. It can help in eliminating the tumor and thus decrease the total amount of drug that must be administered to the patient, thereby reducing the treatment side effects. Mathematically, the influence of the IS corresponds to the addition of a new differential equation $\dot{r}(t)$, where r is the immunocompetent cell density related to various types of immune cells, which influences the tumor volume differential equation through the addition of a new term $-\theta V r$, where θ is a constant coefficient and V is the tumor volume. The total expression of the tumor volume differential equation, considering also the effect of the treatment, is thus

$$\begin{cases} \dot{V}(t) = aV\left(1 - \frac{V}{K}\right) - uV - \theta V r, \\ \dot{r}(t) = \alpha(1 - \beta V)Vr + \gamma - \delta r, \end{cases} \tag{5.10}$$

where u is the treatment effect on the tumor. Figure 5.12 represents the solutions found to be optimal with and without the influence of the immune system.

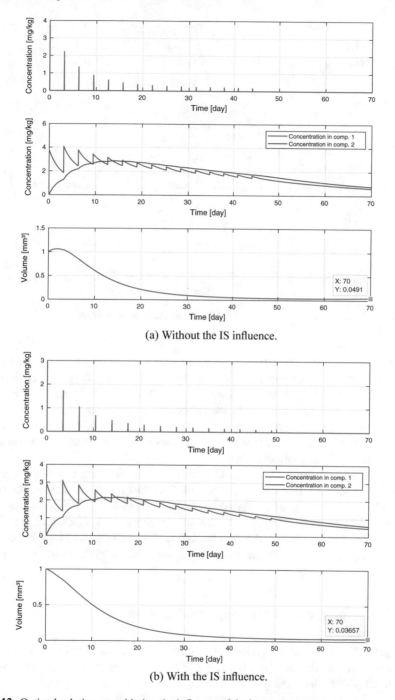

(a) Without the IS influence.

(b) With the IS influence.

Fig. 5.12 Optimal solutions considering the influence of the immune system

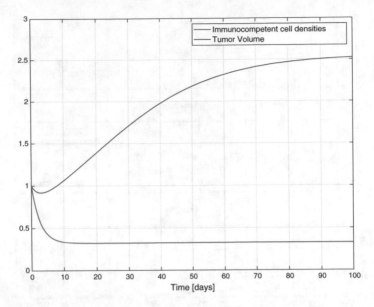

Fig. 5.13 Relationship between the tumor volume and the immune system

One can verify that the IS helps in reducing the tumor volume time evolution. This effect is apparent in the first 10 days of treatment. After that, the tumor evolution is quite similar to that in which the influence of the IS is not considered. This happens because there is also an influence of the tumor on the IS, as one can see in the system of differential equations (5.10). This influence is more noticeable in Fig. 5.13, where the immunocompetent cell densities and the tumor volume are represented without consideration of the treatment effect $u(t)$.

As one may verify in Fig. 5.13, the tumor starts to decrease due to the immune system. Because the immunocompetent cell densities never go to zero, the tumor will not be able to reach its carrying capacity K. This analysis implies that when one considers the immune system, the tumor presents a weaker behavior in terms of growth. This means that the dosages needed in the treatment can be decreased (as Fig. 5.12 suggests), allowing the patient to be less affected by the drug's toxic effect.

5.2.2   Influence of the Angiogenesis Process

The proliferation of cancer cells depends on an adequate supply of oxygen and nutrients. This is why the study of the vascular network is important. As previously stated, angiogenesis is the process by which new blood and lymphatic vessels are formed. Through these new vessels, the tumor obtains the required oxygen and nutrients, and because of that, the angiogenesis process helps the tumor to grow.

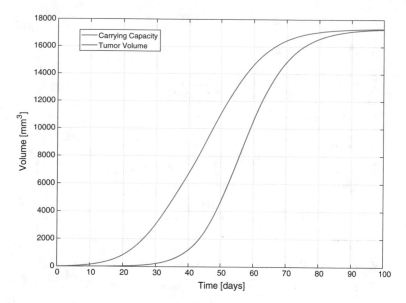

Fig. 5.14 Relationship between the tumor volume and the angiogenesis process

As in the previous section, the angiogenesis process corresponds mathematically to the addition of a new differential equation $\dot{q}(t) = S(V, 1) - I(V, q)$, where q corresponds to the carrying capacity of the tumor. The functions $S(V, q)$ and $I(V, q)$ represent the stimulatory effects that allow the tumor to grow and the inhibitory effects, respectively. These functions can have different expressions. In Enderling and Chaplain (2014) these functions are defined as follows, where the treatment is also considered:

$$\begin{cases} \dot{V}(t) = aV\left(1 - \frac{V}{q}\right) - uV, \\ \dot{q}(t) = \phi V - \varphi q V^{\frac{2}{3}}, \end{cases} \tag{5.11}$$

where ϕ and φ are positive constant rates of angiogenesis stimulation and inhibition, respectively. Figure 5.14 represents the variation of the carrying capacity as well as the tumor volume as described by the differential equations above.

Comparing this behavior with Fig. 3.1, we see that angiogenesis helps the tumor to grow faster. Figure 5.15 represents the solutions found to be optimal with and without the consideration of the angiogenesis process.

As on can see in Fig. 5.15, in order to reduce the tumor, the controller decided to decrease the periodic time interval to increase the amount of drug in the human organism at the beginning of the treatment when the angiogenesis process is considered, because that is the only way to suppress the tumor's growth in the initial phase.

As discussed previously, the immune system helps in tumor reduction, while the angiogenesis process helps the tumor to grow faster. The question now is what

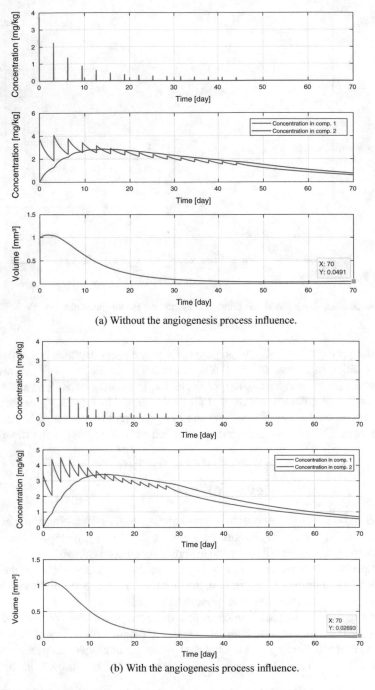

(a) Without the angiogenesis process influence.

(b) With the angiogenesis process influence.

Fig. 5.15 Optimal solutions considering the influence of the angiogenesis process

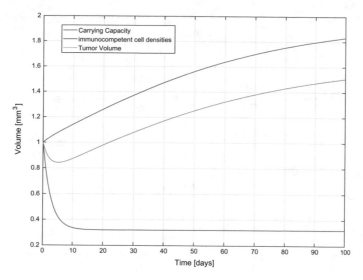

Fig. 5.16 Relationship between the tumor volume, the immune system, and the angiogenesis process

happens when both the IS and the angiogenesis process are considered. This question leads to the system of differential equations

$$
\begin{cases}
\dot{V}(t) = aV\left(1 - \dfrac{V}{q}\right) - uV - \theta Vr, \\
\dot{r}(t) = \alpha(1 - \beta V)Vr + \gamma - \delta r, \\
\dot{q}(t) = \phi V - \varphi q V^{\frac{2}{3}}.
\end{cases}
\tag{5.12}
$$

Figure 5.16 was obtained by simulating the system of equation (5.12). The tumor begins to decrease due to the influence of the immune system, and after that, it begins to increase.

Thus, the optimization problem can be formulated as

$$
\min_{A_1,\dots,A_N,T_p} \int_0^H V^2\,dt + \sum_{n=1}^N \omega_n A_n^2 + \eta_N e^{-T_p+\tau}
\tag{5.13a}
$$

subject to

$$
\omega_n = \alpha\omega_{n-1}, \quad \omega_0 = \rho,
\tag{5.13b}
$$

$$
T_n = T_p, \quad n = 1, \dots, N-1,
\tag{5.13c}
$$

$$
T_p > 0, \quad A_n \geq 0, \quad n = 1, \dots, N,
\tag{5.13d}
$$

$$
\dot{c} = Ac + b\sum_{n=1}^N A_n\delta(t - t_n), \quad T_n = t_{n+1} - t_n,
\tag{5.13e}
$$

$$
u = u_{\max}\frac{c_2}{c_{50} + c_2},
\tag{5.13f}
$$

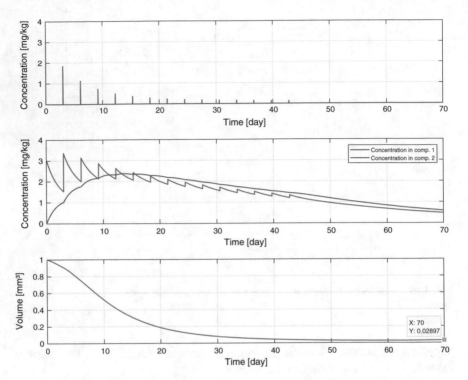

Fig. 5.17 Optimal solutions considering the influence of the angiogenesis process and the immune system

$$\dot{V} = aV\left(1 - \frac{V}{q}\right) - uV + \theta Vr, \ V(0) = V_0, \qquad (5.13\text{g})$$

$$\dot{r} = \alpha(1 - \beta V)Vr + \gamma - \delta r, \qquad (5.13\text{h})$$

$$\dot{q} = \phi V - \varphi q V^{\frac{2}{3}}. \qquad (5.13\text{i})$$

The above optimization problem was solved with ten different initial conditions, and the solution found to be optimal is represented in Fig. 5.17.

As one may observe, the impulse amplitudes are greater than those represented in Fig. 5.12b, where only the influence of the IS is considered, and less than those represented in Fig. 5.15b, where only the influence of the angiogenesis process is considered. Furthermore, the optimal period is less than that represented in Fig. 5.12b due to the influence of angiogenesis, and larger than that represented in Fig. 5.15b, due to the influence of the IS.

Note that for a greater tumor volume, it is necessary to increase the drug concentration, which can be achieved by decreasing the period and increasing the impulse amplitudes, which explains the comparisons in the above paragraph.

5.3   Variable Amplitudes and Time Intervals

In this section, aperiodic and unknown time intervals and amplitudes of the impulses that form the control action are considered. If N is the number of amplitudes, the number of time intervals is $N - 1$. In total, the number of variables in this problem is now $2N - 1$. When this number increases, the number of possible configurations of the variables also increases, which means that the objective function could have more flat areas and local minima, leading to a more complex problem that is not convex. Under these conditions, the optimization problem considered is the following:

$$\min_{A_1,\dots,A_N,T_1,\dots,T_{N-1}} \int_0^H V^2 \, dt + \sum_{n=1}^N \omega_n A_n^2 \tag{5.14a}$$

$$\text{subject to} \quad \omega_n = \alpha \omega_{n-1}, \ \ \omega_0 = \rho, \tag{5.14b}$$

$$T_n > 0, \ \ n = 1, \dots, N-1, \tag{5.14c}$$

$$A_n \geq 0, \ \ n = 1, \dots, N, \tag{5.14d}$$

$$\dot{c} = Ac + b \sum_{n=1}^N A_n \delta(t - t_n), \ \ T_n = t_{n+1} - t_n, \tag{5.14e}$$

$$u = u_{\max} \frac{c_2}{c_{50} + c_2}, \tag{5.14f}$$

$$\dot{V} = aV\left(1 - \frac{V}{K}\right) - uV, \ \ V(0) = V_0. \tag{5.14g}$$

As in the previous section, if small time intervals between impulses are not penalized, the controller will choose them in order to minimize the area under the tumor volume curve, since with this choice, with small intervals and high amplitudes, the drug concentration increases in both compartments. The new terms added in the last section can be also implemented in this problem, but now each time interval will have its own associated weight and exponential or quadratic function. Besides those solutions, a new objective function is considered, where the main goal now will not be minimizing the area under the tumor volume curve but minimizing the final value of the tumor volume.

5.3.1   Minimum Attention Control

As stated at the beginning of Sect. 5.2, the problem of choosing the number N of impulses and the time intervals T_n between them is what makes the optimization problem more complex. If N and T_n are known, then the adjustment of the amplitudes is simple, as Sect. 5.1 suggests. In this section, the concept of minimum attention control is applied in order to understand how N and T_n can be determined, or at least in order to specify an optimization problem that is simpler to solve (Donkers et al. 2011).

In many cases, controllers are still implemented in a time-triggered form, meaning that the control task is executed periodically, in which case the theory of sample data systems can be used. However, overutilization (i.e., a large amount of work handled by a computer) of hardware can occur, since it might not be necessary to execute the control task every period. This leads to the development of several control strategies to reduce computational and communications resources to execute control tasks. Minimum attention control (MAC) is one of those strategies, in which the objective is to minimize the attention the control loop requires. The attention that a control loop requires can be interpreted as the inverse of the sampling time, such that if the sampling time is low, then the controller attention is high (i.e., the controller has to be more frequently active to execute the tasks), and conversely. In other words, MAC maximizes the next time instant in which an impulse is applied, while guaranteeing a certain level of closed-loop performance (Donkers et al. 2011). Therefore, the MAC problem is to find a function F_{MAC} and a function h such that $A_n \in F_{MAC}(c(\sum_{i=0}^{n} T_i))$ and $T_{n+1} = T_n + h(c(\sum_{i=0}^{n} T_i))$, where T_n corresponds to the time intervals between consecutive impulses and the values of $c(T_n)$ correspond to the drug concentrations in both compartments at the time instant $\sum_{i=0}^{n} T_i$ for $n = 1, \ldots, N$, with $T_0 = 0$.

As previously stated, when the time intervals are also considered to be variable, the objective function becomes nonconvex. This fact motivates an investigation into separating the optimization of the amplitudes from the calculation of time intervals. Different ways to reach this objective are considered hereinafter:

- constant areas $\xi_n \cdot A_n \cdot T_n$, where ξ_n corresponds to different weights applied to each area;
- time intervals depending on the tumor volume evolution $T_n \propto \log(V(t_{n+1})) - \log(V(t_n))$, where t_n corresponds to the time instant n of the administration;
- a different objective function for the time instants and another for the amplitudes.

The control is optimized using a certain combination of time intervals. When one of the above methods is used to calculate the time intervals, the amplitudes will no longer be optimal, since the time intervals have changed. Even in considering an iterative approach, no equilibrium between the optimization of the amplitudes and the calculation of the time intervals is reached. Therefore, the strategy to find an optimal solution is the following: the amplitudes and time intervals are optimized together using ten different initial points in the optimization algorithm. The local minimum that yields the minimal objective function value is then chosen.

The adaptation of the MAC concept to the optimal impulsive cancer therapy design problem is simple, since the control task corresponds to the Dirac impulses, and what is needed is to maximize the time intervals between them, maintaining a certain performance that corresponds to tumor volume minimization.

It is known that the tumor volume integral term in the objective function (independently of being the integral either of V^2 or of $|V|$) will force the concentration to increase when the volume is high, which consequently increases the amplitudes and decreases the time intervals. The goal is thus to find a way to maximize the time intervals in such a way that when the tumor volume decreases, the intervals increase. This can be done using, once more, the exponential penalization $\Phi(T_n) = e^{-T_n + \tau}$ or any other function that penalizes small time intervals.

In the case that $|V|$ is penalized, the cost functional for MAC is

$$J(A, T) = \int_0^H |V|\, dt + \sum_{n=1}^N \omega_n A_n^2 + \sum_{n=1}^{N-1} \Phi(T_n), \quad c \in \Omega_c, \tag{5.15}$$

where $\Phi(T_n)$ with $n = 1, \ldots, N-1$ corresponds to any function that penalizes the intervals between consecutive impulses as a function of each time interval. Figure 5.18 represents the optimal solutions for exponential penalization

$$\Phi(T_n) = e^{-T_n + \tau}, \tag{5.16}$$

in Fig. 5.18a, penalization according the function

$$\Phi(T_n) = e^{T_n - (T_n^C + \delta_T)} + e^{-T_n + (T_n^C - \delta_T)}, \tag{5.17}$$

where T_n^C is the point at which the function is minimal and δ_T dictates how close the exponentials are (Fig. 5.18b), negative linear penalization

$$\Phi(T_n) = -T_n, \tag{5.18}$$

in Fig. 5.18c, and also negative quadratic penalization

$$\Phi(T_n) = -T_n^2, \tag{5.19}$$

in Fig. 5.18d, for $N = 10$ administrations and time horizon $H = 70$ days. We remark that the pair of exponentials grow faster than a quadratic function centered at T_n^C. We note as well that each pair of exponentials are centered at different increasing values $T_{i+1}^C > T_i^C$.

The penalty function (5.17) can be compared to the function $\Phi(T_n) = (T_n - T_n^C)^2$. The main difference is that the function with the pair of exponentials yields a higher penalization when T_n is far from T_n^C. Figure 5.19 illustrates this fact. Moreover, Fig. 5.19 also illustrates the behavior of (5.17) for different values of δ_T. As one can see, the parameter δ_T dictates how close the exponentials are. When δ_T decreases, the exponentials approximate, maintaining the minimum of the function, T_n^C. Overall, the penalization for the pair of exponentials is higher than for the quadratic penalization. Furthermore, when we consider the pair of exponentials only, it is also possible to tune how high or low the penalization can be by changing the δ_T parameter. Note, for instance, that for $\delta_T = -1.5$, the value of $\Phi(T_n)$ for $T_n = 12$ is greater than for

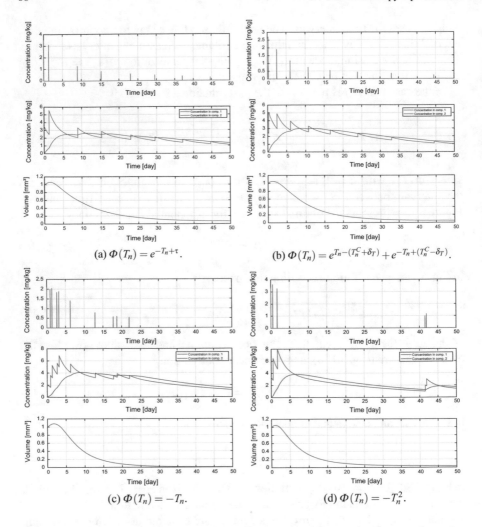

Fig. 5.18 Optimal solutions for exponential, pair of exponentials, negative linear, and negative quadratic penalty functions with constant weights. The integral of $|V|$ and the sum of squared amplitudes in the objective function are also considered

$\delta_T = 0$, and also greater than the quadratic function $\Phi(T_n) = 30 \cdot \left(T_n - T_n^C\right)^2$, for the same instant $T_n = 12$.

We note that because there is no constraint on the maximum value that the intervals can take, the situation $\sum_{n=1}^{N-1} T_n > H$ can occur. In other words, it is possible to have Dirac impulses that do not appear during the treatment session. This fact leads to the variation of the total number of administrations N. As can be seen in Fig. 5.18a, it is possible to count only eight administrations, and in Fig. 5.18b, nine administrations, when actually the initial number of administrations was $N = 10$. If a weight is

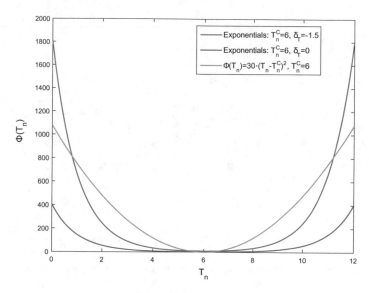

Fig. 5.19 Comparison between the pair of exponentials and quadratic penalty functions for different values of δ_T

added to the penalty function $\Phi(T_n)$, it can work as a tuning knob in terms of the number of administrations N^a that corresponds to the number of impulses such that $\sum_{n=1}^{N^a-1} T_n = H$. If the weight increases, then $N^a < N$, and if the weight decreases, then $N^a = N$, never going higher than the number of administrations N defined initially.

As previously stated in Sect. 5.1.3, the weights applied to each of the impulse amplitudes need to be different in order to penalize the amplitude of the initial impulses more than the later ones, due to the fact that the minimization of the area under the tumor volume curve needs more drug in the first administrations than in the last. From another perspective, the later amplitudes have less impact on the area under the curve. To counteract this effect, a decay rate of 10% in the weights applied was introduced. When the time intervals are also manipulated variables, the same issue arises. That is why in Fig. 5.18, the first time intervals are very small, even when they are penalized by the exponential or quadratic functions. One possible way of defining the weights is by saying that they depend only on the tumor volume at the time instant that the administration is applied. For instance, the weight applied to the first time interval T_1 corresponds to a function $\eta(V(T_1))$; the weight applied to the second time interval T_2 corresponds to a function $\eta(V(T_1 + T_2))$, and so on.

The question now is how this function can be defined. Recall that its main goal is to provide a higher weight when the tumor volume is high and a lower weight when the tumor volume is low. Any function that fulfills this goal can be used. The simplest function is the linear function

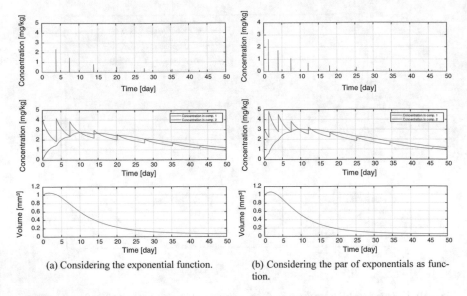

(a) Considering the exponential function.   (b) Considering the par of exponentials as function.

Fig. 5.20 Optimal solutions for both exponential and a pair of exponential functions with linear weights

$$\eta_i \left(V \left(\sum_{n=1}^{i} T_n \right) \right) = a V \left(\sum_{n=1}^{i} T_n \right) + b, \tag{5.20}$$

where η_i corresponds to the weight applied to the exponential or quadratic penalty function of the time interval T_i, $\Phi(T_i)$, and a and b are constant parameters of the linear function. Figure 5.20 represents the solutions found to be optimal for the functions defined in (5.16) and (5.17) as time intervals penalty functions and also for linear weights.

Comparing Fig. 5.20 with Fig. 5.18, we observe that the first time intervals are now increased. In general, what is important to retain is that the weight applied to the penalty function, if it is either constant or described by a linear dependence on the tumor volume, works like a tuning button of the number of administrations N considered during the treatment duration: if the weight increases (in the linear case, if the parameter b increases), N decreases and conversely.

We also note that the integral term in the objective function forces the intervals to be small. In order to introduce the MAC concept in this problem, a penalty function is added, which will force the intervals to be at their greatest possible values, reaching an equilibrium between the integral term and the penalty function. This equilibrium can be tuned by changing the weight η_i. Therefore, the objective function expression for minimum attention control becomes

$$J(A, T) = \int_0^H |V|\, dt + \sum_{n=1}^N \omega_n A_n^2 + \sum_{n=1}^{N-1} \eta_n \Phi(T_n), \quad c \in \Omega_c, \tag{5.21}$$

with Φ as in (5.16) or (5.17) and η_i as in (5.20).

5.3.2 Selection of the Number of Impulses

Previously, the total number of impulses, N, was chosen a priori. In this section, the impact of this choice is discussed.

In the previous section, $N - 1$ time intervals between impulses were considered, where small values were penalized by a function in the cost functional being minimized to yield the optimal control. This penalization leads to an indirect variation of the total number of administrations considered for treatment. There is a simple way of imposing that all the administrations must be inside the treatment period considered. This procedure consists in the addition of one more time interval: the interval T_N between the time horizon H and the time instant of the last administration. With this new variable, is possible to add a new constraint to the optimization problem (as is done in Sakode and Pahi 2018), which is

$$\sum_{n=1}^N T_n = H. \tag{5.22}$$

Since the controller looks at all time intervals equally, this constraint will force the controller to choose an optimal solution in which the time intervals are more evenly distributed in the time horizon H. This requirement means that it is not necessary to use a penalty function in the cost. Establishing a minimum value for the time intervals $T_n^{\min}$ as a constraint in the optimization problem, of $T_n^{\min} = 0.25$ days and optimizing the objective function without any penalty function on the time interval, the solution represented in Fig. 5.21 was found to be optimal, considering also the integral of the absolute value of the volume in the objective function, with $C_{\min} = 0$ and $C_{\max} = 10\,\text{mg/kg}$, as

$$J(A, T) = \int_0^H |V|\, dt + \sum_{n=1}^N \omega_n A_n^2, \quad c \in \Omega_c, \quad \sum_{n=1}^N T_n = H. \tag{5.23}$$

As one can see, even without any interval penalization, the solution has increasing intervals when the tumor size decreases, similar to a minimum attention behavior.

Since the intervals are now better distributed in time (due to the restriction), let us now consider changes in the objective function, in order to obtain some different results, using different perspectives. So far, the mathematical model considered in this work has been adapted to the patient, a time horizon and weights (for the objective

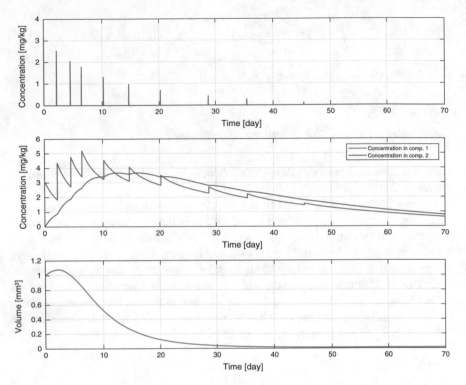

Fig. 5.21 Optimal solution with restriction (5.22)

function) are chosen, and the controller yields the optimal solution that minimizes the tumor volume time evolution and the drug dosages.

Let us consider now that instead of minimizing the tumor volume time evolution, what is minimized is the final tumor volume $V(H)$. The objective function thus becomes

$$J(A, T) = V(H) + \sum_{n=0}^{N-1} \omega_n A_n^2, \quad c \in \Omega_c, \quad \sum_{n=1}^{N} T_n = H. \tag{5.24}$$

We remark that the weights ω_n were added to the impulse amplitudes in order to give each amplitude its own importance and to balance the amplitude values from $t = 0$ to $t = H$. Otherwise, the first amplitudes would have a higher value than the others. This is caused by the integral term in the objective function, since it represents the area under the curve, which is greater at the beginning of the therapy. However, when considering the minimization of the final tumor volume, instead of the entire volume since the beginning of the therapy, this effect (where the first amplitudes have higher values than the others) on the amplitudes may not occur. Therefore, the weights ω_n no longer need to be variable, and thus $\omega_n = \rho$, where ρ is a constant parameter. The objective function becomes

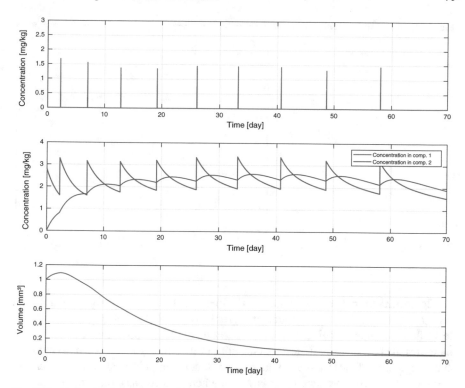

Fig. 5.22 Optimal solution for the objective function presented in Eq. (5.25)

$$J(A, T) = V(H) + \rho \sum_{n=1}^{N} A_n^2, \quad c \in \Omega_c, \quad \sum_{n=1}^{N} T_n = H. \qquad (5.25)$$

Figure 5.22 represents the solution found to be optimal for the above objective function, with $N = 10$ administrations, $C_{max} = 10\,mg/kg$, $C_{min} = 1.5\,mg/kg$, $\rho = 0.003$, and $H = 70$ days. On comparing this figure with Fig. 5.21, we observe that the intervals are now more evenly distributed, since what is important to minimize is the volume's final value instead of the volume's behavior over time. This solution shows better distributed impulses along the time horizon H, which lead to a more constant drug concentration over time in the human organism, as well as a lower average of the concentration, which is an important desideratum for reducing side effects.

Let us now consider a different perspective, in which, besides minimizing the final tumor volume and the amplitudes, the tumor volume evolution is also minimized, leading to the following objective function:

$$J(A, T) = V(H) + \rho \sum_{n=}^{N} A_n^2 + \Psi \int_0^H V\,dt, \quad c \in \Omega_c, \quad \sum_{n=1}^{N} T_n = H. \qquad (5.26)$$

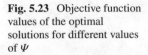

Fig. 5.23 Objective function values of the optimal solutions for different values of Ψ

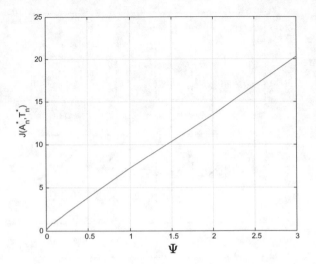

Figure 5.23 represents the value of the objective function in the optimal solution (A^*, T^*) as a function of the parameter Ψ, for $\Psi \in [0, 3]$. As Ψ increases, the importance that the controller gives to the minimization of the tumor volume evolution also increases. It is expected that the drug concentration in the organism begins to increase at the beginning of the treatment, which means that the impulses' amplitudes increase and the tumor's final volume decreases. So, when Ψ increases, the amplitudes will also increase, which explains the behavior of the curve in the above figure.

Figure 5.24 represents the variation of the behavior of the tumor's volume during the treatment (represented by the integral $\int_0^H V\, dt$) and the tumor volume's final value as a function of the parameter Ψ. As one may verify, when Ψ increases, both tumor volume during the optimization time interval and its final value decrease.

Let us consider now a different perspective, whereby the main objective is to minimize the impulse amplitudes subject to the constraint $V(H) = V^*$, where V^* corresponds to a certain desired final tumor volume value, along with the other constraints. This situation corresponds to a scenario in which the objective is to impose a final tumor volume, while minimizing the drug dosages. The objective function is now the following:

$$J(A, T) = \rho \sum_{n=0}^{N-1} A_n^2, \quad c \in \Omega_c, \quad \sum_{n=1}^{N} T_n = H, \quad V(H) = V^*. \tag{5.27}$$

Set $\rho = 1$. Note that the objective function is now convex, due to the fact that it corresponds to a linear combination of convex functions. However, the problem as a whole is not convex. The problem here is to satisfy the constraint $V(H) = V^*$. Figure 5.25 represents the solution found to be optimal for the problem in (5.27).

Because now the goal is to have a specific final tumor volume value, there are many different possible configurations that can achieve that goal.

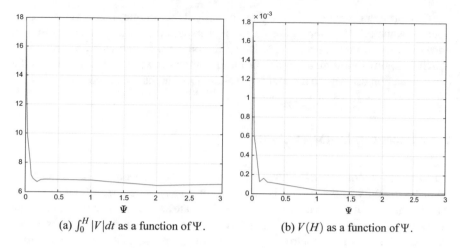

(a) $\int_0^H |V|dt$ as a function of Ψ.

(b) $V(H)$ as a function of Ψ.

Fig. 5.24 Behavior of the tumor's volume during treatment and its final value, for the optimal solutions for different values of Ω

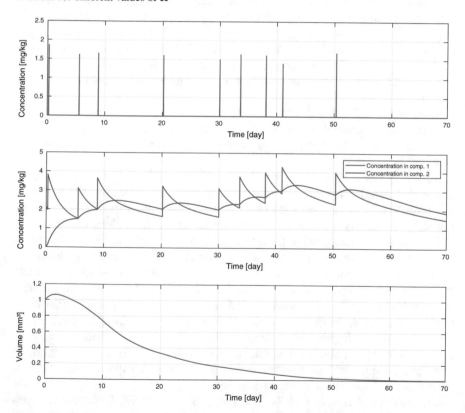

Fig. 5.25 Optimal solution for the objective function presented in (5.27)

If the problem were to minimize the tumor's final volume, the number of con-figurations would be lower. However, in this perspective, it was possible to find an objective function that is convex, reducing the problem to one with constraints for which an optimization method such as the IP method can be used, since it uses the barrier function concept to maintain the solution inside the feasible area.

5.4 Receding Horizon Control

Up to now, the control law found has been an open-loop one. The sequence of impulses to apply to the patient is designed for a fixed time span H, and depends only on the patient's state at initial time. Future states are computed using this state only and the mathematical model of cancer evolution. If a disturbance causes a state deviation, the open-loop control law is unable to compensate for these deviations.

The most common way to obtain a closed-loop control law from an optimal open-loop control law is to resort to the receding horizon control (RHC) strategy. Accordingly, only the first impulse i of the optimal impulse sequence computed between $t = t_i$ and $t = t_i + H$, where t_i are the time instants at which the drug is administrated as defined in Sect. 1.2, for $i = 1, \ldots, N$, is applied at the time instant t_i, the whole process being repeated for the interval of time between $t = t_{i+1}$ and $t = t_{i+1} + H$, starting from the state at $t = t_{i+1}$, this procedure being repeated in sequence.

Using the receding horizon strategy, the patient's state is used to generate a sub-optimal feedback control action every t_i samples, for $i = 1, \ldots, N$. In Lemos et al. (2016) this strategy has been studied in relation to the control of tumor growth in myeloma bone disease.

Applying this concept to the problem of this work, the following is done: for a finite horizon $0 \leq t \leq H$, solve the OIC problem and select just the first drug administration to be applied to the patient; next, move the time horizon into the future, for instance $t_2 \leq t \leq H + t_2$, and solve the new OIC problem, where the new initial conditions correspond to the final conditions of the previous OIC problem at $t = t_2^-$; repeat the procedure (iterate the procedure) by moving the time horizon.

Figure 5.26 illustrates the RHC process for three iterations. In iteration two, there is one drug administration already selected for the treatment, and the OIC problem corresponds to $0^2 \leq t \leq H^2$, where 0^i and H^i are the time horizon limits for itera-tion i. In the figure, the dislocation time ΔH is $\Delta H = T_n$, with $T_n = $ constant for $n = 1, \ldots, N - 1$. Depending on the shift time parameter, the number of selected drug administrations at each iteration can vary. When ΔH increases, the number of selected administrations also increase, which means that the receding horizon evolves faster. However, this is not necessarily good.

For instance, if $\Delta H > T_1 + T_2$, the number of selected administrations at each iteration is $\#s^i = 2$. This means that a new piece of information is added to the OIC problem in every two time intervals, which can lead to more sudden changes in

Fig. 5.26 Receding horizon illustration of three iterations, with $N = 4$

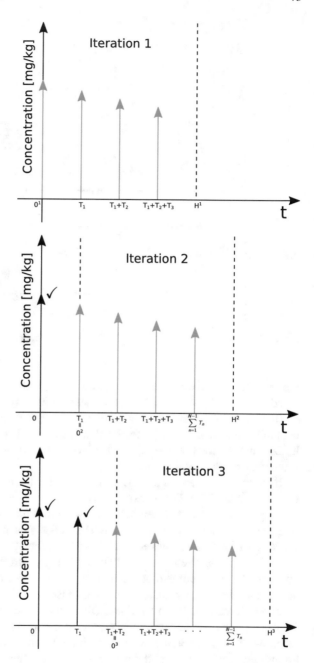

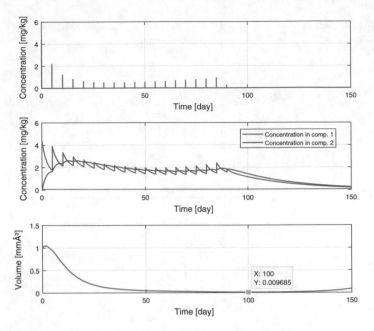

Fig. 5.27 Optimal solution for $H = 150$, $N = 30$, $T_p = 5$, and $\rho = 0.3$

the selected administrations. If the tumor increases between two time intervals, the receding horizon control will adapt to that change only after two administrations.

Because each selected drug administration has more information about the tumor evolution, this technique adds feedback to the optimal controller. Each time the time horizon moves, the previous optimal solution readapts to the new information, even if the tumor suddenly increases.

In order to compare RHC to OIC, it is possible to simulate the model considered in this work as Fig. 5.27 suggests.

As previously stated, when the tumor volume is too small, the controller chooses to decrease the amplitudes, since their impact is almost null in the volume evolution. Besides that difference between RHC and OIC, the other difference is in the amplitudes themselves. The reason for that is that the controller does not know anything about the future tumor evolution. Indeed, it is possible to see that at the end of the simulation, the tumor volume starts to increase again.

The difference between RHC and OIC can be made clearer in the face of disturbances. A disturbance can be introduced in the model in many different ways: by resetting the tumor volume integrator with a different initial condition, introducing an instantaneous change in the tumor volume; by changing the maximum effect of the drug in the tumor by changing the u_{max} parameter of the PD model, as stated in Sect. 3.5; or even by changing any other parameter of the total model described in Sect. 3.5.

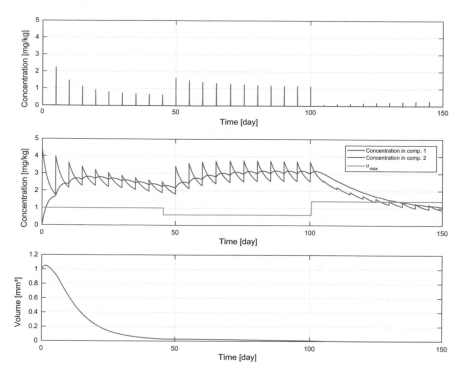

Fig. 5.28 Receding horizon control simulation, with changes in the parameter u_{max} as perturbation

In a real-world scenario, resetting the integrator with different initial conditions corresponds to an instantaneous increase in the tumor volume during the treatment that cannot be a real phenomenon. On the other hand, changing the maximum effect of the drug in the human organism can model a real situation: at a certain period of the treatment, the human organism could react differently to the drug, causing different effects in the tumor, for the same drug concentration. Figure 5.28 represents the RHC applied to the model with this perturbation occurring twice, at $t = 45.5$ and $t = 100.5$ days, where for $t \in [0, 45.5[$, $u_{max}(t) = 1$, for $t \in [45.5, 100.5[$, $u_{max}(t) = 0.6$, and for $t \in [100.5, 150]$, $u_{max}(t) = 1.4$. It is also considered that the value of ρ decreases 10% at each iteration of the RHC procedure $\rho^k = 0.9 \cdot \rho^{k-1}$, $\rho^1 = 0.3$, where k is the RHC iteration, ρ being kept constant for all of the impulses of each OIC problem.

For $t \in [45.5, 100.5[$, the drug has less effect on the tumor volume, so the RHC increases the amplitudes to compensate for the loss of effect. For $t \in [100.5, 150]$, the drug has greater effect on the tumor volume, and the RHC decreases the amplitudes to reduce the unnecessary side effects of the drug.

Now Fig. 5.29 is obtained by simulating the model using the OIC method without the RHC strategy. As one can see, the OIC cannot adjust the solution to the perturbations, because it does not have feedback, in contrast to RHC.

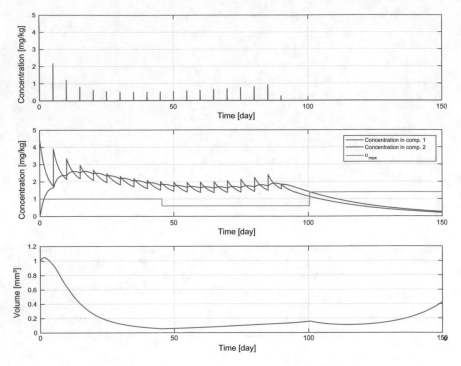

Fig. 5.29 Optimal impulsive control simulation with changes in the parameter u_{max} as perturbation, without the RHC strategy

References

Anderson B, Moore JB (1969) Linear system optimization with prescribed degree of stability. Proc IEE 166(12):2083–2087

Donkers MCF, Tabuada P, Heemels WPMH (2011) On the minimum attention and the anytime attention control problems for linear systems: a linear programming approach. In: 50th IEEE conference on decision and control and European control conference, Orlando, USA

Enderling H, Chaplain MAJ (2014) Mathematical modeling of tumor growth and treatment. Curr Pharm Des 20(30):4934–4940

Lemos JM, Caiado DV, Coelho R, Vinga S (2016) Optimal and receding horizon control of tumor growth in myeloma bone disease. Biomed Signal Process Control 24:128–134

Sakode CM, Pahi R (2018) Nonlinear impulsive optimal control synthesis with optimal impulse timing: a pseudo-spectral approach. IFAC J Syst Control 3:30–40

Chapter 6
Complementary Aspects

6.1 Sensitivity Analysis

There are two possible approaches to modeling parameter sensitivity analysis, one relying on analytical methods and the other, used here, that resorts to simulations in which the controller designed for the nominal value of the model parameters is coupled to the plant model in which the parameters have been perturbed.

Another aspect of sensitivity analysis is concerned with the impact of variations of the parameters that define the controller on the resulting performance.

6.1.1 Parameter Variation

The controller relies on the model described in Sect. 3.5, where the objective function is

$$J(A, T) = \int_0^H |V| \, dt + \sum_{n=0}^{N-1} \omega_n A_n^2, \quad c \in \Omega_c, \quad \sum_{n=1}^N T_n = H, \qquad (6.1)$$

where $C_{min} = 1.5$ mg/kg, $C_{max} = 10$ mg/kg, and $H = 70$ days.

The parameters considered in this section are the initial tumor volume value $V(0)$, the maximum effect of the drug concentration u_{max}, and the carrying capacity of the logistic model K. These parameters are considered because they have greater impact on the controller's performance. In the previous chapter the parameter values considered were $V(0) = 1$ mm^3, $u_{max} = 1$, and $K = 5$. The optimal solution obtained from these values is presented in Fig. 6.1.

When changing the initial tumor volume to $V(0) = 5$ mm^3 while maintaining the other parameters constant, the optimal solution is as shown in Fig. 6.2.

Comparing Fig. 6.2 to the solution presented in Fig. 6.1, higher amplitudes would be expected here, since the initial volume is greater. However, note that now

J. P. Belfo and J. M. Lemos, *Optimal Impulsive Control for Cancer Therapy*,
SpringerBriefs in Control, Automation and Robotics,
https://doi.org/10.1007/978-3-030-50488-5_6

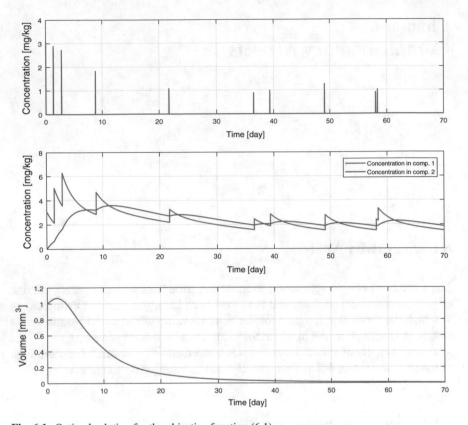

Fig. 6.1 Optimal solution for the objective function (6.1)

$V(0) = K$, which means that the tumor is at its maximum volume. In other words, if no treatment is considered, the volume derivative is zero, according to the logistic equation. This means that when the treatment is applied, the tumor will start to decrease immediately, allowing the amplitudes to be small.

For $V(0) = 3\,\text{mm}^3$, the optimal solution is the one shown in Fig. 6.3. We observe that the previous situation does not occur. Since the derivative of the volume is not zero for $t = 0$, the drug concentration in the period $0 \le t \le 10$ days is greater than the concentration in the simulation shown in Fig. 6.2 for the same period, even for a lower initial volume. One may conclude that treating a tumor that is already at its maximum size requires less drug concentration at the beginning of the treatment for this particular case.

As explained in Sect. 5.1.3, the amplitude weights ω_n are proportional to the initial volume. This detail is important for the balance between the integral term and the amplitudes term in the objective function. Figure 6.4 represents the same situation described above, except that the amplitude weights are not proportional to the initial volume.

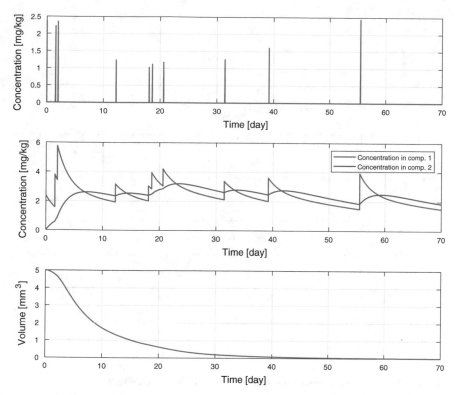

Fig. 6.2   Optimal solution for the objective function (6.1), for $V(0) = 5\,\text{mm}^3$

One can see that the amplitudes are now allowed to be higher, since their penalization weight has decreased. Because of that, the time intervals are also allowed to have greater values, since the drug concentration can be increased by the drug dosages (amplitude values).

The solution found to be optimal for the parameter configuration $u_{max} = 0.5$, $V(0) = 1\,\text{mm}^3$, and $K = 5$ is represented in Fig. 6.5.

Because the drug concentration now has less impact on the tumor's evolution, the amplitudes were forced to increase in order to minimize the tumor volume. However, because of the amplitudes' weights, the maximum concentration restriction was not reached. An equilibrium between minimizing tumor volume and toxicity effect was reached. This study can be used to test new drugs for improved performance during treatment.

Increasing the drug's maximum effect to $u_{max} = 1.5$ leads to the optimal solution represented in Fig. 6.6.

As one may verify, the amplitudes have decreased, and the time intervals have, on average, a greater value compared to the situation in which $u_{max} = 0.5$. This comparison shows that the variation of this parameter can substantially influence the optimal solution, allowing a better solution in terms of attainability and toxicity. The

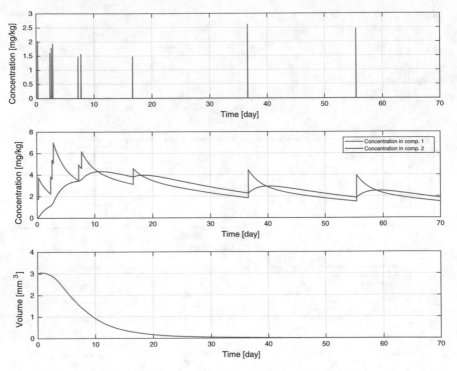

Fig. 6.3 Optimal solution for the objective function (6.1), for $V(0) = 3\,\text{mm}^3$

impulse amplitudes did not present lower values due to the minimum concentration restriction $C_{\min} = 1.5\,\text{mg/kg}$.

Take now $K = 10\,\text{mm}^3$ while maintaining the other parameters at their original values. The optimal solution is represented in Fig. 6.7.

Comparing this solution with the solution presented in Fig. 6.1, one can verify that the impulse amplitudes have higher values in this solution than in the solution in Fig. 6.1. This is due to the fact that when K increases, the volume derivative also increases, since the difference between $V(0)$ and K also increases (recall the logistic equation (3.2)).

6.1.2 Modeling Errors

In this section, the behavior of the controller solution is studied when there are errors in model parameters with respect to their nominal values. Such errors correspond to the same parameters previously considered: $V(0)$, $u_{\max}$, and K. In order to analyze the controller's behavior, it is necessary to define a criterion that can describe the performance of an optimal solution of a certain problem when those parameters are

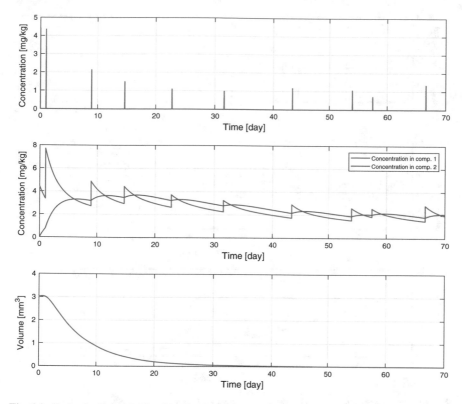

Fig. 6.4 Optimal solution for the objective function (6.1), for $V(0) = 3\,\text{mm}^3$, for amplitude weights not proportional to the initial volume

not those on which the controller was based. The chosen criterion corresponds to the time evolution $\int_0^H |V|\,dt$ of the tumor volume and the tumor's final volume $V(H)$.

The results in Fig. 6.8a and b are obtained for the optimal solution presented in Fig. 5.21 and change in the parameter $V(0)$. As one may verify, using the same optimal solution when the initial volume is smaller than the original (which is $1\,\text{mm}^3$), both tumor volume time evolution $V(t)$ and its final value $V(H)$ decrease, and conversely. Furthermore, both curves suggest that there is a certain error value from which the variation in both tumor volume time evolution $V(t)$ and its final value $V(H)$ decrease, suggesting a saturation. We observe that the tumor carrying capacity remains constant at $K = 5\,\text{mm}^3$. So when the initial volume satisfies $V(0) < K$, the volume derivative is positive, meaning that the tumor has not reached its maximum volume, and as previously stated, the controller will have to compensate for the fact that it needs first to force the derivative to zero and then become negative, leading to an increase in the amount of drug administered. When $V(0) = K$, the derivative is zero, meaning that the tumor has already reached its maximum value (the controller just needs to force the derivative to be negative). For $V(0) > K$, the derivative is

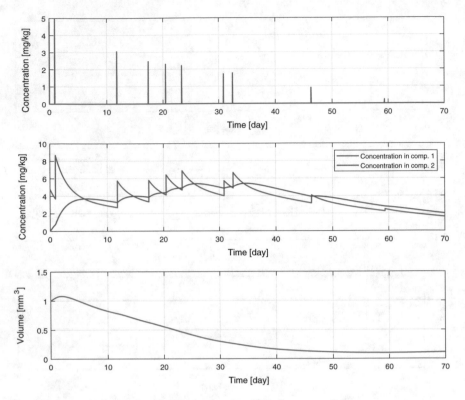

Fig. 6.5 Optimal solution for the objective function (6.1), for $u_{max} = 0.5$

already negative, meaning that the tumor volume is greater than its final equilibrium value (in this situation, the amount of administered drug is much less than in the previous situations). So when the error is equal to four (meaning that the initial volume is equal to five), the derivative changes its sign to a negative value. This is why both curves decrease.

Considering now the variation of the parameter u_{max}, the tumor volume integral and final value depend on the error, as shown in Fig. 6.9.

The parameter u_{max} corresponds to the maximum effect that a certain drug concentration has on the tumor. When this parameter increases, the same amount of drug has a greater effect on the tumor's evolution, leading to a decrease in both tumor volume evolution $V(t)$ and the final value $V(H)$. As previously stated, it is also possible to verify in Fig. 6.9b that increasing the treatment effect in the tumor does not lead to a zero tumor final volume.

For the variation of the parameter K, the tumor volume evolution and final value behave as shown in Fig. 6.10. When K increases, the initial volume derivative also increases, since the difference between the initial volume and its maximum value (final value) increases. The behavior is similar to that shown in Fig. 6.9.

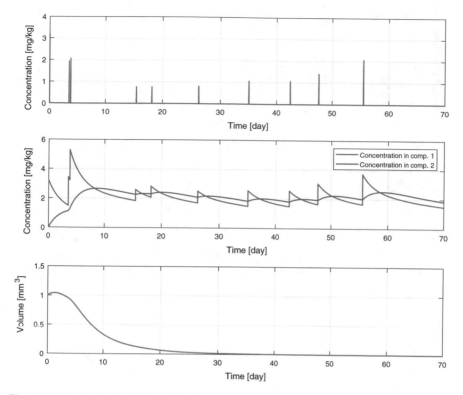

Fig. 6.6 Optimal solution for the objective function (6.1), for $u_{max} = 1.5$

6.1.3 Quantization

In this section, the effect of quantization on the control variables is considered. In other words, the values of the control variables are quantized using different resolutions. For instance, if the resolution is 0.5, the control variables can only have values that are multiples of 0.5.

In order to study the impact of quantization, the optimal solution considered in Fig. 5.21 is again used, and its objective function is evaluated for different quantization values. What is actually happening is that when the quantization increases, a value that is really $A_1 = 2.643$, for instance, becomes $A_1 = 2.60$ when the quantization is 0.05, $A_1 = 2.5$ when the quantization is 0.5, and so on. So the quantized value decreases when the quantization increases. This means that the amplitudes and time intervals will start to decrease. Recall that the objective function considered penalizes only the amplitudes. Because the amplitudes decrease, due to the quantization, the objective function value in the optimal solution also decreases. However, when the amplitudes decrease, there will be less drug administered, which could increase the tumor volume evolution (leading to an increase in the integral term). But the time intervals also decrease, which will allow the accumulation of drug in the human

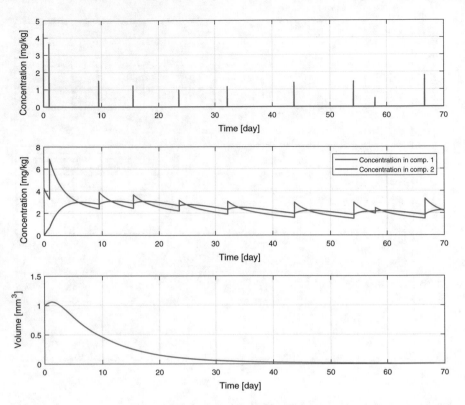

Fig. 6.7 Optimal solution for the objective function 6.1, for $K = 10$

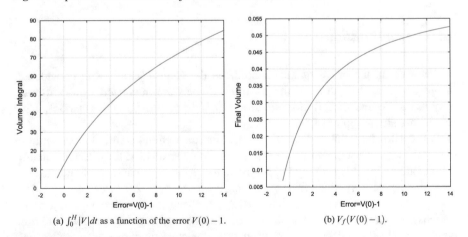

(a) $\int_0^H |V| dt$ as a function of the error $V(0) - 1$.

(b) $V_f(V(0) - 1)$.

Fig. 6.8 Tumor volume time evolution and tumor final volume as functions of the error $V(0) - 1$, where $V(0) \in [0.4, 15] \, \text{mm}^3$ and the value 1 corresponds to the initial volume used for the optimal solution

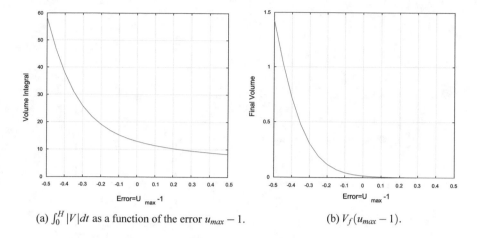

(a) $\int_0^H |V|\,dt$ as a function of the error $u_{max} - 1$.

(b) $V_f(u_{max} - 1)$.

Fig. 6.9 Integral of tumor volume and tumor final value as functions of the error $u_{\max} - 1$, where $u_{\max} \in [0.5, 1.5]\,\text{mm}^3$ and the value 1 corresponds to the initial $u_{\max}$ value used for the optimal solution

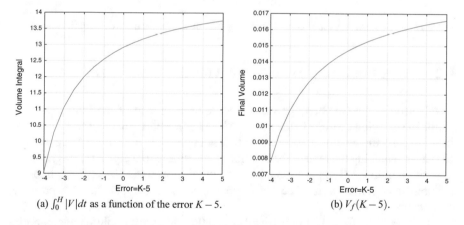

(a) $\int_0^H |V|\,dt$ as a function of the error $K - 5$.

(b) $V_f(K - 5)$.

Fig. 6.10 Tumor volume time evolution and tumor final value as functions of the error $K - 5$, where $K \in [1, 10]\,\text{mm}^3$ and the value 5 corresponds to the initial value of K used for the optimal solution

organism, leading to a decrease in the tumor volume. And so in the end, the objective function's value in the optimal solution decreases, as shown in Fig. 6.11, due to the decrease in the amplitudes.

Figure 6.12 represents the original optimal solution and the solution for a quantization of 1 in the control variables. Note that the tumor volume evolution is almost the same for both the original and quantized solutions.

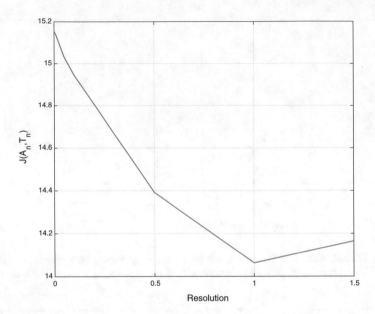

Fig. 6.11 The objective function considered in Fig. 5.21 evaluated for different quantization values

6.2   Using the Gompertz Growth Model

In this section the Gompertz growth model is used instead of the logistic model. While the carrying capacity in the logistic model corresponds to the K parameter, in the Gompertz model, the carrying capacity is not explicit in the differential equation. However, by taking the limit of the solution of the differential equation, it is possible to verify that in the Gompertz model, the carrying capacity is $K_G = V_0 e^{\frac{a}{b}}$. In order to compare both models, it is necessary to parameterize them such that they have the same carrying capacity.

For $K = 5$, $V(0) = 1$, $a = 0.1$, and $b = 0.062$, the tumor volume evolution in time for both models is as shown in Fig. 6.13. As one may observe, for these parameters, the curves for both models are very similar. However, we note that the curve in Fig. 6.13a reaches its final value faster than the curve in Fig. 6.13b. Using those same parameters and using constant time intervals $T_n = 3$ days for $n = 1, \ldots, N - 1$, the optimal solutions for both models are represented in Fig. 6.14.

It is remarked that a higher value of the drug concentration is required when the Gompertz model is used. Observing the curves in Fig. 6.13, we see that in the beginning, the tumor's growth using the Gompertz model is faster than that computed with the logistic model. For $10 < t < 20$, the growth is faster using the logistic model, which occurs only when the volume is between 2 and 3 mm^3. When treatment is considered, such growth does not occur. So the reason that the drug concentration

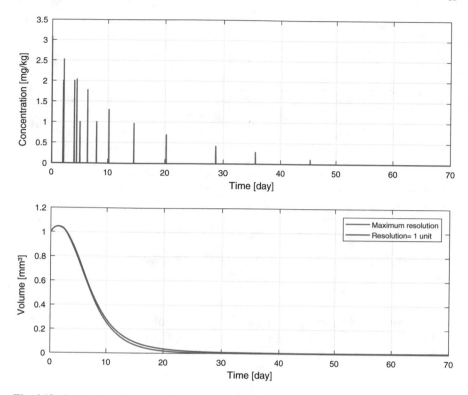

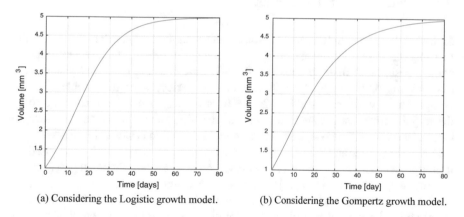

Fig. 6.12 Original solution and solution for a quantization of 1

(a) Considering the Logistic growth model. (b) Considering the Gompertz growth model.

Fig. 6.13 Tumor volume time evolution for both logistic and Gompertz growth models

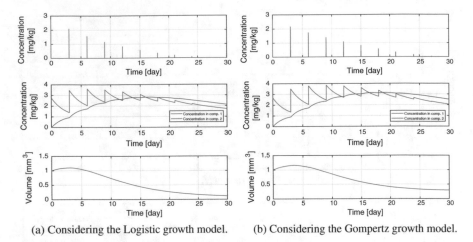

(a) Considering the Logistic growth model.　　(b) Considering the Gompertz growth model.

Fig. 6.14 Optimal solutions for periodic time intervals with period $T_p = 3$, $N = 10$, and $H = 30$ days

is higher with the Gompertz growth model is that for volume values around $1\,\text{mm}^3$, the Gompertz model yields a faster volume growth, forcing the amplitudes of the impulses in the control signal to increase.

6.3　Pseudospectral Methods

So far, we have concluded that what makes the optimization problem difficult is the fact that the impulse time instants can also change in time. In fact, several impulse control design techniques proposed in the literature consider fixed time instants and that only the Dirac impulse amplitudes can be varied, since that problem is less complex to solve (Sakode and Pahi 2018). In order to consider the situation in which the impulse time instants are also treated as decision variables, the need to develop computationally efficient algorithms for model integration is increasing. This issue is discussed in Sakode and Pahi (2018), where a pseudospectral approach is proposed. In this approach, the state variables are represented in terms of orthogonal polynomials of time, where the idea is to project the nonlinear high-dimensional state variables (in the general case) onto a finite low-dimensional problem that is easier to solve. In other words, the optimal control problem solution is projected onto a low-dimensional nonlinear problem solution by the selection of grid points at which the solution is forced to be exact, and then this problem is solved using a computationally efficient optimization algorithm.

The fact that the pseudospectral method requires a low number of grid points leads to a low-dimensional optimization problem, which yields a faster method than those used above.

There are several different polynomials that can be used for this purpose. For instance, Chebyshev polynomials with Chebyshev–Gauss–Radau (CGR) or Chebyshev–Gauss–Lobatto (CGL) grid points can be used.

In order for this technique to be applied, first the problem needs to be rewritten in terms of a normalized time, whereby each time value must be in the interval $[-1, 1]$, where -1 corresponds to the initial time instant and 1 corresponds to the final time instant.

Chebyshev polynomials are given by $\phi_N(\tau) = \cos(N \cos^{-1}(\tau))$, where N is the degree of the polynomial, $\tau = \cos(\theta)$, $\tau \in [-1, 1]$ and $\theta \in [0, \pi]$. So the first terms of the polynomial are $\phi_0(\tau) = 1$, $\phi_1(\tau) = \tau$, and the next terms are given by the recurrence

$$\phi_{N+1}(\tau) = 2\tau\phi_N(\tau) - \phi_{N-1}(\tau). \tag{6.2}$$

The corresponding relationship in differential form is given by

$$\dot{\phi}_{N+1}(\tau) = 2\phi_N(\tau) + 2\dot{\phi}_N(\tau) - \dot{\phi}_{N-1}(\tau). \tag{6.3}$$

Considering, for instance, the CGR grid points, the $N + 1$ points are given by $\tau_c = \cos(\frac{\pi c}{N})$ for $c = 0, 1, 2, \ldots, N$. Note that the computation of the grid points and the polynomials is fast due to the existence of the recurrence relationships.

Next, in the objective function, the state differentiation is approximated by taking the differentiation of the approximating polynomials

$$x_{iq}^{\tau} \approx \sum_{k=0}^{N-1} a_{iq}^k \phi_k(\tau), \quad \dot{x}_{iq}^{\tau} \approx \sum_{k=0}^{N-1} a_{iq}^k \dot{\phi}_k, \tag{6.4}$$

where x_{iq}^{τ} is the ith state variable at the qth interval for the normalized time τ, N is the number of Chebyshev polynomials used to approximate the state variables, and a_{iq}^k is the weight applied to the polynomial k of the segment q of the state variable i. In matrix form, the nonlinear system $\dot{X} = f(X)$, where f is a nonlinear function of the state vector $X = [x_1, \ldots, x_i]$, can be written as

$$A_q\dot{\phi}(\tau_c) = \frac{\Delta T_q}{2} f(A_q\phi(\tau_c)), \text{ for } \tau_c \in (-1, 1), \tag{6.5}$$

with the jump condition

$$A_q\phi(-1) = g(A_{q-1}\phi(+1), u_q), \tag{6.6}$$

where the term $\frac{\Delta T_q}{2}$ appears from the time normalization in each q interval, A_q is the weight matrix, and $\phi(\tau_c)$ corresponds to the vector of polynomials. These two equations correspond to constraints of the optimization problem, along with the constraint on the intervals $\sum_{q=1}^{S_q} \Delta t_q = t_f$, $\Delta t_q \geq 0.25$ and the impulse amplitude constraint $C_{max} = 10$ and $C_{min} = 1.5$ mg/kg. See Sakode and Pahi (2018) for more details.

In the model considered in this work, there are two state variables: concentration in compartment one, c_1, and in compartment two, c_2. However, the objective to optimize is the minimization of tumor volume. Here we propose to add one more state, which corresponds to the tumor volume V, that depends on c_2, which in turn depends on c_1. The three states are needed for the formulation of the optimization problem. The main idea here is to approximate each of the three states using N weighted Chebyshev polynomials. By approximating the states, the differentiation of the states is done by the differentiation of the polynomials. The weights, which are also optimization variables, are chosen such that the differential equality is maintained. The time intervals and the impulse amplitudes are also optimization variables. The parameters needed to be defined correspond to the total number of administrations and the number of polynomials used to approximate the states.

Figure 6.15 represents the solution found for 10 administrations and 10 Chebyshev polynomials and the constraints already considered in the above optimizations, along

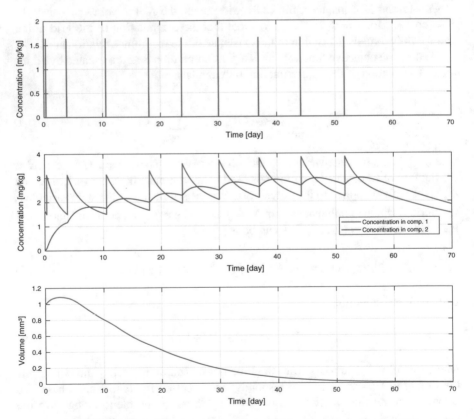

Fig. 6.15 Optimal solution using a pseudospectral method for the objective function presented in Eq. (5.25)

with the final tumor volume constraint $V(H) \leq V^*$. This solution is similar to the solution presented in Fig. 5.22, since the aim is to minimize the impulse amplitudes and also the tumor volume, even if this last goal is inserted in the constraints, in addition to finding the right polynomials weights. The computational time used for the optimization algorithms to find the optimal solution of this problem is relatively less than the time used for the other problems. This feature is due to the fact that what is being solved does not correspond to the real problem but to an approximation. If the number of polynomials used increases, then in the limit, there will be no difference between the real and the approximate problems, and they will each take the same amount of time.

As previously stated, in order to find the best solution, the optimization problem is solved using ten different initial points, and then the solution that gives the lowest objective function is considered the best solution (among all ten solutions). For the parameter configuration used for finding the solution presented in Fig. 6.15, all ten solutions were exactly the same.

Reference

Sakode CM, Pahi R (2018) Nonlinear impulsive optimal control synthesis with optimal impulse timing: a pseudo-spectral approach. IFAC J Syst Control 3:30–40

Chapter 7
Conclusions and Research Topics

7.1 Conclusions

This book addresses the problem of optimizing cancer therapy using optimal control methods. The distinguishing feature is that *the control (manipulated) variable is a train of Dirac impulses* for modeling therapeutic actions that are concentrated in specific time instants, such as the ingestion of pills.

Although impulsive optimal control is, in general, a very difficult subject, the assumption that the control variable affects the model in a linear way, and that an a priori known number of impulses is used, allows one to reduce the control design problem to a *finite-dimensional optimization problem* that can be tackled with a convenient solver, a feature explored in this book.

The solution of the basic optimal control problem associated with cancer therapy yields an open-loop control law that is unable, without any modification, to compensate for the effect of model errors and disturbances. In order to obtain a feedback control law, the basic optimal control sequence is used in a *receding horizon strategy* that amounts to applying to the patient only the first control action of the sequence and repeating the whole dynamic optimization procedure starting from the patient's state at the next discrete time instant. The advantage of this approach, tightly related to model predictive control for impulsive systems, is demonstrated in the presence of disturbances.

The innovative approach to cancer therapy suggested and demonstrated in this book relies on the concept of *minimum attention control*. This strategy suggests adjusting the time between consecutive control impulses according to the patient's state. To this end, the cost function is suitably modified to allow for optimization with respect to the time interval between successive impulses, as well as the impulse amplitudes. As a result, the number of impulses per unit time (a measure of the controller's "attention") is greater than when the tumor size is smaller.

The main content of this book is organized as follows: Chap. 2 begins with the study of compartmental models as pharmacokinetic models. The Hill equation is used

J. P. Belfo and J. M. Lemos, *Optimal Impulsive Control for Cancer Therapy*,
SpringerBriefs in Control, Automation and Robotics,
https://doi.org/10.1007/978-3-030-50488-5_7

as a pharmacodynamic model, which introduces a saturation in the concentration of two-compartmental evolution.

Chapter 3 studies two tumor growth models: logistic and Gompertz. Each of them introduces a saturation effect in the tumor volume evolution. Two subsystems that influence the tumor volume evolution are presented: immune system and angiogenesis. These subsystems are modeled by extra states whose dynamics also depend on the tumor volume. The immune systems begin to attack the tumor, reducing the volume. Because the immune system is also affected by the tumor, its strength also decreases, leading to an equilibrium in which the tumor will continue to grow, depending on the initial tumor volume and the initial immunocompetent cell densities related to various types of immune cells (T-cells). The angiogenesis process represents the variation of the tumor's carrying capacity in time, which allows the tumor to grow faster and to reach a much greater volume, which also depends on the initial volume, carrying capacity, and some other parameters.

Chapter 4 shows how to approximate the solutions of the optimal impulsive control problem associated with cancer therapy by the solutions of a finite-dimensional nonlinear programming problem.

Chapter 5 applies this method, first with a periodic sequence of impulses and then with an aperiodic one, according to a minimum attention control strategy. In order to obtain a feedback solution, a receding horizon control strategy is followed.

Chapter 6 addresses some relevant complementary issues, including the sensitivity of control to parameters and quantization, the use of the Gompertz growth model instead of the logistic model, and a model discretization with a pseudospectral method.

7.2   Research Topics

The following are open research topics:

1. *Using more elaborate cancer models.* This book considers a number of cancer dynamic models, with a model for tumor growth coupled with other physiological subsystems that affect it, such as the immune system and angiogenesis. More detailed models of these, and other, subsystems can be considered. Since increasing the number of model states and model complexity yields a larger computational load for control action optimization, a point to clarify is the best compromise between model complexity and control performance. Modeling for control is, however, not just a matter of computational complexity, and capturing the underlying physiological mechanisms is a major issue. For this reason, considering classes of cancer (for instance, bone marrow cancer) will provide interesting specializations of controller design.

2. *Multitherapy design.* The main ideas are illustrated in this book only for therapy with a single agent. When several drugs, or therapeutic agents, are considered, what is their optimal combination? In addition to centralized optimization, the

design of therapies based on distributed control agents may also be envisaged, with these agents cooperating according to distributed optimization methods derived from game theory or distributed alternating direction method of multipliers (D-ADMM). In some situations, the use of multitherapy implies the consideration of different administration rates, a problem that may be tackled with the methods from multirate control or hierarchical control. Some therapies may evolve continuously in time, as well as impulsive control actions. This hybrid control problem requires appropriate laws that can be derived by applying numerical methods to versions of the maximum principle for impulsive optimal control (Miller and Rubinovich 2003; Arutyunov et al. 2019). An in-depth knowledge of impulsive optimal control is thus required.

3. *Models with a nonlinear dependency on the control variable.* In this case, obtaining the optimal impulsive control may not be reduced to a finite-dimensional problem by the use of simple properties of distributions, and one has to resort to the theory of impulsive optimal control. Of course, an issue to consider at the outset is to show the advantage of cancer models for which the control variable enters in a nonlinear way.

4. *Adaptive control.* A major problem faced in designing controllers for physiological systems is the large uncertainty associated with interperson variability, as well as with the same person under different circumstances. This high level of uncertainty can be tackled with the methods of adaptive control. Although there are several approaches to adaptation, a suitable one is supervised multiple model adaptive control, in which different possible models are compared, in real time, with the actual observed patient behavior in order to find the best match (Teles and Lemos 2019). The selected model, which also depends on a dwell-time condition to prevent instability associated with fast switching, is then used to compute the control action. Although other approaches are possible to enable adaptations in control, such as certainty equivalence or explicit criterion minimization, the use of supervised multiple models is quite appealing, because this method allows one to explicitly include, right from the design stage, known possibilities with physiological significance. Another promising approach is nonlinear adaptive control, relying on reinforcement learning and adaptive dynamic programming (Lewis and Vrabie 2009), for which impulsive optimal control raises new challenges.

5. *State estimation.* This book has concentrated on control design and makes the simplified assumption that the state variables are available for direct measure, which, of course, is not realistic. The design of appropriate state estimators is thus an important issue that must take into consideration the impulsive character of the input. In addition to control variable computation, state estimators are also important to detect abrupt changes in dynamics, as well as to tackle the situation in which output measurements are not available at all time instants, requiring their estimation. Although other approaches are possible, one based on moving horizon estimation (Goodwin et al. 2005) appears to be a natural choice to handle the impulsive inputs.

6. *Nonideal impulses*. Modeling concentrated therapy actions by Dirac impulses is just one approximation. This approximation is better than assuming that the control is given by a continuous time function, but it is not exact. A question is thus what the impact on the overall system performance will be if the actual therapy actions are not exactly Dirac impulses.

7. *Properties of receding horizon impulsive control*. The properties of receding horizon control are well known, both for linear and nonlinear systems (Kwon and Han 2005) when the manipulated variable is a continuous function of time. In particular, the enforcement of constraints that ensure stability or turnpike properties (Trélat and Zuazua 2015) for large horizon values are well studied, although in some cases, they remain the subject of research. There is not yet a complete theory establishing corresponding properties for receding horizon impulsive control.

8. *Other forms of minimum attention control*. As previously explained, minimum attention control is likely to play a major role in the control of physiological systems. This approach has been illustrated in this book using a particular formulation of the cost function being optimized. A research topic is to extend the implementation of minimum attention control using different costs and to other situations, such as multitherapy. In effect, one may consider the situation in which several drugs are used, each with a different time constant for action, thereby demanding multirate control or event-driven control, a topic currently receiving much attention (Newzari et al. 2019; Proveda et al. 2019).

9. *Continuous drug effect control and impulsive therapy control*. There are many published studies that take as manipulated variable the drug effect, which is a continuous variable. When the therapy is applied through impulsive actions, how can these two actions be made compatibile? One possibility might be a cascade control architecture, in which the designed (continuous) drug effect is approximated by an impulsive controller. If this approach is followed, what is its effect on optimality?

10. *Application to other diseases*. The treatment of other diseases also employs impulsive actions, an example being HIV infections (Pinheiro et al. 2011). As such, the techniques described in this book may as well be applied to other such cases.

References

Arutyunov A, Karamzin D, Pereira FL (2019) Optimal impulsive control. Springer, Berlin
Goodwin GC, Seron M, De Doná JA (2005) Constrained control and estimation. Springer, Berlin
Kwon WH, Han S (2005) Receding horizon control. Springer, Berlin
Lewis FL, Vrabie D (2009) Reinforcement Learning and adaptive dynamic programming for feedback control. IEEE Circuits Syst Mag 9(3):32–50
Miller BM, Rubinovich EY (2003) Impulsive control in continuous systems. Springer Science+Business Media, LLC, Berlin

Newzari C, Garcia E, Cortés J (2019) Event triggered communication and control of networked systems for multi-agent consensus. Automatica 105:1–27

Pinheiro JV, Lemos JM, Vinga S (2011) Nonlinear MPC of HIV-1 infection with periodic inputs. In: 50th IEEE conference on decision and control and European control conference, Orlando, Fl, USA, pp 65–70

Proveda JI, Benosman M, Teel AR (2019) Hybrid online learning control in networked multiagent systems: a survey. Int J Adapt Control Signal Process 33(2):228–261

Teles FF, Lemos JM (2019) Cancer therapy optimization based on multiple model adaptive control. Biomed Signal Process Control 48:255–264

Trélat E, Zuazua E (2015) The turnpike property in finite-dimensional nonlinear optimal control. J Differ Equ 258:81–114

Series Editor Biographies

Tamer Başar is with the University of Illinois at Urbana-Champaign, where he holds the academic positions of Swanlund Endowed Chair, Center for Advanced Study (CAS) Professor of Electrical and Computer Engineering, Professor at the Coordinated Science Laboratory, Professor at the Information Trust Institute, and Affiliate Professor of Mechanical Science and Engineering. He is also the director of the Center for Advanced Study—a position he has held since 2014. At Illinois, he has also served as interim dean of engineering (2018) and interim director of the Beckman Institute for Advanced Science and Technology (2008–2010). He received the B.S.E.E. degree from Robert College, Istanbul, and the M.S., M.Phil., and Ph.D. degrees from Yale University. He has published extensively in systems, control, communications, networks, optimization, learning, and dynamic games, including books on noncooperative dynamic game theory, robust control, network security, wireless and communication networks, and stochastic networks, and has current research interests that address fundamental issues in these areas along with applications in multiagent systems, energy systems, social networks, cyber-physical systems, and pricing in networks.

In addition to his editorial involvement with these briefs, Başar is also the editor of two Birkhäuser series, *Systems & Control: Foundations & Applications* and *Static & Dynamic Game Theory: Foundations & Applications*, the managing editor of the *Annals of the International Society of Dynamic Games* (ISDG), and member of the editorial and advisory boards of several international journals in control, wireless networks, and applied mathematics. Notably, he was also the editor-in-chief of *Automatica* between 2004 and 2014. He has received several awards and recognitions over the years, among which are the Medal of Science of Turkey (1993); Bode Lecture Prize (2004) of IEEE CSS; Quazza Medal (2005) of IFAC; Bellman Control Heritage Award (2006) of AACC; Isaacs Award (2010) of ISDG; Control Systems Technical Field Award of IEEE (2014); and a number of international honorary doctorates and professorships. He is a member of the US National Academy of Engineering, a Life Fellow of IEEE, Fellow of IFAC, and Fellow of SIAM. He

© The Author(s), under exclusive license to Springer Nature Switzerland AG 2021
J. P. Belfo and J. M. Lemos, *Optimal Impulsive Control for Cancer Therapy*,
SpringerBriefs in Control, Automation and Robotics,
https://doi.org/10.1007/978-3-030-50488-5

has served as an IFAC advisor since 2017, a Council Member of IFAC (2011–2014), president of AACC (2010–2011), president of CSS (2000), and founding president of ISDG (1990–1994).

Miroslav Krstic is Distinguished Professor of Mechanical and Aerospace Engineering. He holds the Alspach endowed chair, and is the founding director of the Cymer Center for Control Systems and Dynamics at UC San Diego. He also serves as Senior Associate Vice Chancellor for Research at UCSD. As a graduate student, Krstic won the UC Santa Barbara best dissertation award and student best paper awards at CDC and ACC. Krstic has been elected Fellow of IEEE, IFAC, ASME, SIAM, AAAS, IET (UK), AIAA (Associate Fellow), and as a foreign member of the Serbian Academy of Sciences and Arts and of the Academy of Engineering of Serbia. He has received the SIAM Reid Prize, ASME Oldenburger Medal, Nyquist Lecture Prize, Paynter Outstanding Investigator Award, Ragazzini Education Award, IFAC Nonlinear Control Systems Award, Chestnut textbook prize, Control Systems Society Distinguished Member Award, the PECASE, NSF Career, and ONR Young Investigator awards, the Schuck ('96 and '19) and Axelby paper prizes, and the first UCSD Research Award given to an engineer. Krstic has also been awarded the Springer Visiting Professorship at UC Berkeley, the Distinguished Visiting Fellowship of the Royal Academy of Engineering, and the Invitation Fellowship of the Japan Society for the Promotion of Science. He serves as editor-in-chief of *Systems & Control Letters* and has been serving as senior editor for *Automatica* and *IEEE Transactions on Automatic Control*, as editor of two Springer book series—*Communications and Control Engineering* and *SpringerBriefs in Control, Automation and Robotics*—and has served as vice president for technical activities of the IEEE Control Systems Society and as chair of the IEEE CSS Fellow Committee. Krstic has coauthored thirteen books on adaptive, nonlinear, and stochastic control, extremum seeking, control of PDE systems including turbulent flows, and control of delay systems.

Printed in the United States
By Bookmasters